D0849884

Cancer Biology,
A Study of Cancer
Pathogenesis

CANCER BIOLOGY, A STUDY OF CANCER PATHOGENESIS

How to Prevent Cancer and Diseases

Migdalia Arnán, MD

Library of Congress Control Number:		2011960988
ISBN:	Hardcover	978-1-4653-0667-8
	Softcover	978-1-4653-0666-1
	Ebook	978-1-4653-0668-5

It is not intended to serve or as replacement for professional medical advice. Recommendations mentioned in this book are not to be taken without the advise of medical doctors, naturopatic physician, registered dietitian or other specialist.

This book was printed in the United States of America.

To order additional copies of this book, contact:
Xlibris Corporation
1-888-795-4274
www.Xlibris.com
Orders@Xlibris.com
104462

TABLE OF CONTENTS

Hemoglobin transport. Bacteria in cancer tissue. Macrophages and Alpha-fetoprotein. Hemoglobulin and oxygen transport. Blood supply in cancer. Mycoplasma-like bodies in plants and in animal tissues.

Cancer and nutrition.
Immunity and cancer. Infections and cancer. Disproteinemia and immunecomplexes. Localized antigenic stimulation.

Free radicals, Oxygen and ozone.
Experimental effect of ozone in human and in mice cancer cells. Electron photographs demonstrating the effect of ozone on the RBCs of mice with mammary cancer. Electron photograph of RBC of human with cancer of the breast. Effect of light on cancer cells of human and in mice. The Green Granules, (GG). Characteristics of the GG in cancer cells and in macrophages. Electron photograph of quantosome-like body in human ovarian cancer.

Protein molecules tridimentional confirmation. Cell transformation. Molecular changes at the cell surface. Antibody and immuneglobulines composition. Specificity of the antibodies. Immune defence system. Allergy, vaccine and immunity in the pathogenesis of disease. Allergic manifestations. Membrane surface receptors.

The immunologic basis of diseases.
Viral antibodies associated with malignancy. Human tumor viruses. Viral oncogenesis. Immune response in tumor—bearing. T-cells in cancer.

Can fungus be the cause of cancer.
Frequently misdiagnosed skin fungus infection. Treatment of fungus skin infection. Diet for patients with fungus infection. Detoxification and changes in life-style. Diet and life-style for cancer patients.

DEDICATION

This book, Cancer Biology, A Study of Cancer Pathogenesis, is dedicated to the Almighty God, The Creator of the Universe, The Light of the World.

Also,

To the memory of my parents, Luis Arnan Suria and Mercedes Guerra Peres, who impregnated in my mind the importance of knowledge and the need to find answers to the why, who, what and how of situations.

To my sisters, Elive Arnan and Yvette Miller.

To the memory of my husband, David Archibald Morrissey Sanderson who supported me in my work.

To my daughter, Laura Gaebler, and to my grandchildren, David Alexander and Daniel Jackson Gaebler, to my granddaughter Jessica Olive Larson, and to my greatgrandchildren, Quintin, Cooper and Kieran Larson.

I am thankful to the many scientists, who in the quest for the truth, and with their important discoveries, have set basic foundations for those to follow. Without their work, this book would not be possible.

This book is not only intended for medical doctors of all specialties, but also it will be helpful to researchers, biologists, nurses, and to the general public interested in learning and desiring to take an active part in their health.

INTRODUCTION

Cancer has the unique ability to replicate endlessly as long as it has the proper environment. It can grow and infiltrate the adjacent normal tissue, crowding it with overlapping tumor cells. As cancer does not recognize cell boundaries, it stretches its cell-dividing tentacles to suffocate its victims.

Cancer grows at the expense of the patient's healthy tissues. It is an infectious parasitic tumor growth that occurs in genetically predisposed individuals with a decreased immunity, when exposed to specific tumor sensitizers and promoters.

Why are cancer cells so unique, so different from normal cells that make them ageless? Why are cancer cells able to grow uncontrollably? Why are cancer cells unable to recognize cells boundaries? Why are cancer cells so pleomorphic?

Why do cancer cells replicate so effectively? Why do cancer cells have an anaerobic metabolism? What are the fundamental molecular changes that transform a normal cell into a malignant cell?

What is the significance of the "green granules" (GG) found in living cancer cells when exposed to light? Is there any similarity between the metabolism of a cancer cell and a plant cell? Is the cancer cell a proof of the survival of the fittest? What role does the macrophage play in cancer pathogenesis (initiation) and in cancer metastases?

What role does the immune system play in cancer pathogenesis? What is the effect of ozone gas (O_2-O_3) on cancer and on the membrane of the red blood cells (RBCs)?

Can cancer be prevented? Can it be cured?

These and other cancer-related subjects will be addressed in this book.

INTRODUCTION

CHAPTER I

Characteristics of Cancer Cells

Immortality of Cancer Cells. Given the proper nutrition and environment, cancer cells outlive any normal cell. For example, cells from the Rous sarcoma and from the HeLa carcinoma are malignant cells lines kept alive and used in laboratory experiments years after their original host's death.

HeLa cells were isolated by Gey in 1951 from a cell line of an adenocarcinoma of the uterine cervix of a thirty-seven-year-old woman, Henrietta Lacks. Descendents of the original HeLa cell line are still thriving in the laboratory, in tissue cultures throughout the world years after the demise of its original source. Similarly, Ehrlich's ascitic tumor cells originated in 1938 from a solid mouse's tumor and have been kept multiplying in vitro by mouse to mouse transfer. A two-year-old mouse is quite old, but Ehrlich's solid tumor mouse cells are still growing while non-transformed normal cells in culture have a limited number of divisions. This indicates that somatic cells have a specific intrinsic number of divisions compared with the cancer cells.

While spontaneous cancer cells are immortal, this is not the case in carcinogen-transformed cells, whose life span is finite. Thus, immortality is a property of cancer cells, but not of normal or artificially transformed cells.

Cancer Cells Do Not Recognize Cell Boundaries. Normal tissue cells in culture stop growing when in contact with another cell—contact inhibition. Thus, in tissue culture, normal cells form a single cellular layer covering the culture plate surface. Cancer cells, on the contrary, do not recognize cell boundaries piling on top of each other, forming uneven mounds of unruly cellular growth.

Cancer Cells as Unruly Parasites. Cancer cells are programmed for unrestrained growth and to successfully compete for nourishment at the expense of the adjacent healthy tissue. Normal cells, on the contrary, are programmed to work in harmony with each other for the benefit of the whole body. Cancer cells are like the young cowbird, dropped in another bird's nest by the mother, who eats voraciously and often pushes the other young birds out of the nest.

Abnormal Morphology. Cancer cells have a genetic predisposition to heterogeneity, which means they have a variety of forms. Not only is there a variation in size of the cancer cells, but there is also a multi-potential morphologic appearance with a tendency to vary from the original tissue character.

Examination of tissue from various areas of the cancer may show a diversity of cells, cellular patterns, and behavior from the original tumor site. Cancer cells vary from two to ten or more times the size of normal cells. Some of the cancer cells can be multinucleated, even forming giant tumor cells. The chromatin pattern is pleomorphic, hyperchromatic, and bizarre; and usually, there are numerous cells in mitosis (cell divisions). Changes are also noted by electron microscopy. A primitive cellular morphology suggests rapid tumor growth and a more guarded prognosis (poor outcome).

Abnormal Chromosomes in Cancer. Chromosome changes, such as the Philadelphia chromosome (Ph) found in chronic granulocytic leukemia, are usually one and a half to two times larger than normal chromosomes. This and other chromosomal anomalies are used as markers in tumors, in congenital and other diseases. Association of acute leukemia in mongolism is a known fact. However, the incidence of leukemia could be higher if mongols lived longer.

Chromosome anomalies can affect the sex chromosomes as well as the autosomes. Many diseases are now associated with specific chromosome alterations. Chromosome breakage is associated with oncogenic virus infection. It has been stated that if the oncogenic (cancer producing) gene is incorporated into a host genome, (genetic blue print) there will be a continue replication of the oncogenic gene, and tumor growth independent of the initial infection. There is a relationship between chromosome counts and both invation and degree of differentiation in transitional cell carcinoma of the bladder.

Certain human leukemias and lymphomas show specific and consistent chromosome translocations: Chromosome eight is involved with chromosome two, fourteen, or twenty-two. Other anomalies in the translocation between chromosome eight and fourteen. While in myeloid leukemia the long arm of chromosome nine translocates to chromosome twenty-two, but in acute promyyelocytic leukemia, the long arm of chromosome seventeen translocates to chromosome 15.

Karyotype alterations in malignancies of the gastrointestinal tract have been found. The changes affect not only the number of the chromosomes, but the morphology as well.

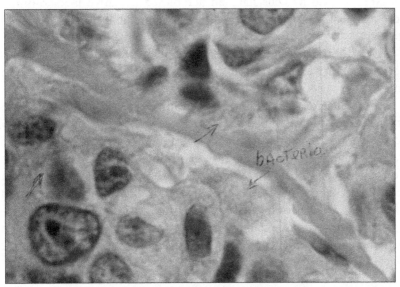

Infiltrating poorly differentiated carcinoma

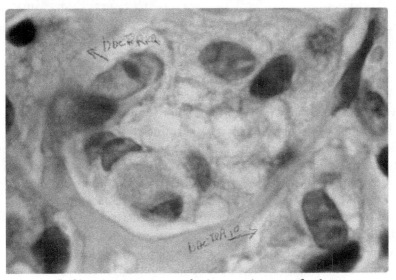

Infiltrating mucus-producing carcinoma of colon

Anaerobic Metabolism of Cancer Cells. Otto Warburg won a Nobel Prize in 1936 because of his discovery of the anaerobic or fermentative metabolism of cancer cells. Normal healthy cells have an aerobic or oxidative metabolism, while cancer cells have an anaerobic or fermentative metabolism. What triggers the metabolic change that transforms a normal cell into a cancer cell?

Because of the ineffective fermentative metabolism of the cancer cells, the cancer cell energy is channeled toward cellular replication instead of having a harmonious and cooperative relationship with other cells and tissues.

It is the anaerobic metabolism of cancer cells that make them susceptible to radiotherapy. During radiation, energy is transferred to electrons which ionize the matter they reach. This ionization also affects the DNA and the RNA by weakening them. Changes are possible due to the recombination of the damaged molecule with the available free O_2 (oxygen) in the environment. The cellular changes produced by the radiation under oxygenated conditions can be fatal to the cell, or it can inhibit cell proliferation. Without the presence of oxygen, the radiotherapeutic effect is impossible. The limiting effect of radiation is dependent upon the degree of vascularization of the tumor. Cancers that have poor vascularization are more radioresistant because there is less oxygen available.

Healthy cells rely on mitochondria for their normal oxidative metabolism. Mitochondria are microscopic spheres or rods found in a cell's cytoplasm. Their number varies from a few to hundreds, depending on the cell's activity. For example, a rat's hepatocyte (liver cell) is a very active cell and may contain one thousand mitochondria.

Altmann first observed and described the mitochondria toward the end of the nineteenth century. A few years later, Benda named them mitochondria, but it was Otto Warburg who associated the mitochondria with respiratory enzymes and therefore with cell respiration.

Examined by electron microscopy, the mitochondria are round or cylindrical bodies enclosed by two membranes. The inner membrane has projections or folds called cristae. These are at the inner membrane level, where formation of adenosine triphosphate (ATP) occurs with oxidation of reduced enzymes and where oxidative phosphorylation occurs. The cristae are more numerous in areas of greatest activity. Mitochondria membranes have a greater amount of lipids than the endoplasmic reticulum membranes.

Cancer cells decrease the number and size of mitochondria. These frequently contain calcium deposits and are ineffective.

Mitochondria in Cancer Cells. There is a marked reduction in the number of mitochondria in tumors with high fermentative or glycolytic rate. Tumor cells grown in a glucose-containing medium may produce large amounts of lactic acid in comparison with the normal control cells. Some tumor cells in vitro use predominantly fatty acids and amino acids, specifically glutamine, as a source of fuel.

Warburg theorized in 1930 that cancer cells have an anaerobic or fermentative metabolism resulting in increased glycolysis. Since the respiratory or oxidative capacity of the cell depends on its mitochondria and its function is inhibited or not present in cancer cells, it is of the utmost importance to study not only the physiology of the normal mitochondrion, but that of the cancer cell as well.

There is a 50 percent or more reduction in the number of mitochondria in rapidly growing tumors. Why? In a rapidly growing tumor, where fast production of nutrients is necessary, why revert to a less-efficient anaerobic metabolism? Is this occurring because nourishment of the cancer cells is already available from the surrounding environment, ready-made for the fast-dividing cancer cells?

Pendersen has reported on the low number of mitochondria in most rapidly growing tumors and on the lower yield of mitochondria from such tumors in comparison with the content in the slow-growing tumors.

Pendersen and others interpreted that the poor respiratory capacity may be "due, at least in part, to the low mitochondrial content rather than to an inhibition of the electron transport chain per se." But not all tumors have abnormal content or deficiency in the electron transport chain as reported by Wallach in 1975. Ruggiere and Falani in 1968 and others have found an increase of cholesterol in tumor mitochondria and that the inner mitochondrial membrane has a higher concentration of cholesterol than the outer membrane.

Hepatoma's (cancer of the liver) mitochondria contain more calcium than a normal hepatocyte (normal liver cell). Calcium inhibits the ATP/ADP (adenosine triphosphate / adenosine diphosphate) translocation step in Ehrlich ascites mitochondria. This would prevent the uptake of ADP and therefore inhibit the synthesis of ATP as demonstrated by Thorne and Bygrave in 1974.

It is possible that the increased levels of intramitochondrial cholesterol are due to the accumulation of metabolic by-products that the mitochondria are unable to burn up due to the deficient oxidative metabolism of the cancer cell. Hence, it accumulates not only in the mitochondria but in the cells as well.

DNA Molecules in Mitochondria.

There are two to six DNA molecules in each mitochondrion. Each DNA molecule is double circular, and each measures about 5_{um} in circumference. In cancer, however, double circular dimers are twice as large as the size of a single circular monomer (10_{um}), which may represent almost 50 percent of the total number of mitochondrial DNA.

Irwin and Malking in 1976 found that two to three proteins synthesized by mitochondria of hepatoma might have a different molecular weight than that synthesized by normal liver mitochondria.

Bass in 1977 found that there was an increased protein synthesis in hepatomas, two to three times as that found in the normal control. These findings imply specific alteration of the cancer's mitochondria coding mechanism as suggested by Pendersen.

What genetic changes, if any, are responsible for the alterations? Are these changes viral related? What significance has the presence of dimers in mitochondria? Where does the extra genetic material come from in order to double the size of the dimers? Is this the result of virus-mitochondrion integration?

However, not all cancers are virus related. How about the cancer induced by radiation or chemicals? Radiation or chemically damaged fragments of the mitochondria DNA could rearrange in such a way that the repaired mitochondria DNA may have an altered physiology capable of taking over the cellular control from the nuclear DNA. Thus, DNA alterations could transform the normal cellular behavior into a cancer physiology.

Mitochondrial Alterations Following Cell Injury. With cell death, there are progressive changes occurring in the mitochondria, such as swelling, accumulation of calcium, and others, including tubular formations. Tubular formations occur as the result of fragmentation of the inner membrane during the later stages of mitochondria degeneration.

Mitochondria Characteristics. Mitochondria are round or sausage-shaped organelles found in the cell's cytoplasm, and they are essential for normal cell functions. Mitochondria have been called the "cell's furnace," where energy is generated through ADP and ATP.

These organelles are enclosed in a double membrane and are more abundant in very active healthy cells. In yeasts grown under anaerobic conditions without a source of fatty acids and sterols, mitochondria are completely absent, or only an occasional single membrane vesicle is observed within the cytoplasm when studied by electron microscopy.

Mitochondria utilize formylmethionine for protein synthesis. The mitochondria enzyme tRNA (transfer ribonucleic acid) polymerase is capable of formylating methionine. This enzyme is different from the polymerase found in the nuclear RNA. Another characteristic of mitochondria is its undergoing of genetic recombination—mitochondria can incorporate genes from other structures. The recombination in mitochondria may be similar to the bacterial plasmid since both have a circular DNA. Initiation and replication of the circular mitochondria DNA may be continuous since the origin and the terminus are adjacent. This form of replication does not need any nuclear or cytoplasmic command; it is independent.

The previous information is of the utmost importance, for it can give us some insight on how cells could divide endlessly if the control of the cell is taken over by the mitochondria instead of the nucleus as normal.

All of the above indicates that mitochondria have a protein-synthesizing ability of their own, independent of the cell cytoplasm-protein synthesis. However, some mitochondria proteins are coded by the nuclear DNA, as in cytochrome C, RNA polymerase, mitochondrial DNA polymerase, and others.

Does cancer initiation occur when specific oncogenic viruses integrate with the mitochondria DNA and thus trigger a metabolic instability or change from the normal cell oxidative to a fermentative or anaerobic metabolism, resembling primitive microorganisms or plantlike physiology?

In normal repairing mitochondria, at physiologic pH, the ATP (adenosine triphosphate) has one more negative charge than the ADP (adenosine diphosphate). This charge is transported into the extramitochondrial space, but in the "presence of uncouplers which negate the membrane potential this presence of the ATP efflux is cancelled."

If the circular DNA of the mitochondria becomes impregnated by the circular DNA of an acceptable virus, the biological instability provoked by such an occurrence may very well precipitate a reverse electron transfer. Such a reverse electron transfer may create difficulty in the production of ATP, and thus, the oxidation potential is reduced. This will produce accumulation of cellular wastes, and instead of eliminating cholesterol and formic acid, formaldehyde (HCHO) is produced and retained. Formaldehyde, a known growth promoter and a carcinogenic, may stimulate the cell into a constant division. Thus, an endless division cycle may be initiated.

In 1965, Somlo and Fukuhara reported that the synthesis of mitochondrial cytochromes in saccharomyces only occurs in the presence of oxygen. Whether other mitochondrial constituents are present in anaerobically grown cells, it is dependent on the growth medium chosen. Numerous well-defined mitochondria-like structures are present when the culture medium is supplied with a source of sterols and fatty acids.

It has been reported that at a very high glucose concentration, there is a marked fermentation, and the biosynthesis in mitochondria is almost completely repressed and that all the cytochromes are in very low concentrations. When fermentation is low because the sugar concentration is low or because other sugars are used as carbon source (for example, melibiose, which cannot be fermented by saccharomyces), respiration may be as high as that of cells grown on lactate.

May it be extrapolated from above that a diet rich in refined carbohydrates could stimulate a fermentative cellular metabolism and thus act as a cancer promoter development and growth? Since sugar predisposes fermentation, could this, together with a viral infection, alter the cell's metabolism and transform it from the normal oxidative to the fermentative metabolism of the cancer cell?

With fermentation, there is inhibition of the normal mitochondria respiration and biosynthesis; and therefore, there is less ATP available for the normal oxidative metabolism. Thus, anaerobic metabolism occurs.

The most important function of mitochondria is the oxidative phosphorylation, whereby energy is released via ADP/ATP during electron transfer.

The mitochondria DNA are represented by a circular dimer, the size of which varies from the largest in plants to the smallest in man.

Protein Synthesis in Mitochondria. Mitochondria have all the required elements for protein synthesis. It utilizes N-formylmethionine as the initiating amino acid. Chloroplasts (plant organelle containing little bodies called quantosomes, essential for photosynthesis) resemble mitochondria in its independent protein-synthesizing ability.

The Mitochondria DNA. The mitochondria is the only other part of the cell besides the nucleus to have DNA in a double helix. But it is a circular DNA similar to the circular bacterial DNA. Mitochondria may have several DNA molecules. Some of the plant mitochondria may have more DNA information and are larger than the animal mitochondria. There is genetic information suggesting that the hereditary characteristic of mitochondria depends on the mitochondrial genes and mitochondrial cytoplasmic factors.

Plant and animal mitochondria divide and replicate. This observation has been made with phase microscopy and confirmed by electron microscope studies. Neurospora, a mold's variant, cannot synthesize choline, a prominent component of cell's membrane phospholipids. Based on this, D. Luck carried experiments with neurospora growing in a medium containing labeled choline. He demonstrated the doubling in the number of the mitochondria after culturing it for several hours.

Isolated mitochondria have an avidity for calcium with subsequent granules enlargement and an increase in electron opacity. In pathologic conditions, mitochondria may have inclusions in the form of crystals and filaments. Intramitochondrial crystals have been observed in livers of normal pregnant women and in women under steroid or oral contraceptives.

Yeasts grown in an oxygenated environment show an oxidative metabolism with the presence of cytochrome and regularly appearing mitochondria. But when exposed to an anaerobic media, there is almost complete absence of cytochromes. Studies by electron microscope show few double bodies with scarce internal structures and rare, if any typical, mitochondria. This returns to normal with the return to an oxygenated environment.

What do all of the above have to do with cancer? If cancer has a fermentative metabolism, what changes are present in the cancer cell's mitochondria and/or any other part of the cell to account for the cell's metabolic change?

Mitochondria with normal rapid oxidative metabolism behave as the furnace of the cell. It depends on the normal production of ATP for oxidation and elimination or neutralization of cellular wastes. How is the formation of ATP in cancer cells inhibited or altered?

Erythrophagocytic Ability of Cancer Cells. In my laboratory, I have observed that cancer cells engulf red blood cells (RBCs). By microscopic examination of over five hundred hemathoxylin and eosin (H&E) stained sections of different kinds of cancers, I have found that 10 percent of the cancer cells contained RBCs, either intact or partially fragmented. This erythrophagocytic ability of cancer cells was noted in all cancers studied such as cancer of the skin, breast, lung, stomach, uterus, cervix, prostate, and in one case of leiomyosarcoma of the leg.

Greenfield and Price found high iron content in and around neoplasms by using isotope-labeled RBCs. However, when they utilized tagged-hemolyzed RBCs, no iron deposits were found. Their data suggest that the intact RBCs were deposited directly into the tumor.

My observation of the erythrophagocytic ability of the cancer cell (cancer cells engulf red blood cells) not only supports their findings but also explains it. During digestion of the RBCs by the cancer cells, the iron content of the hemoglobin is retained by the cancer cells and surrounding tissues (connective tissue or macrophages).

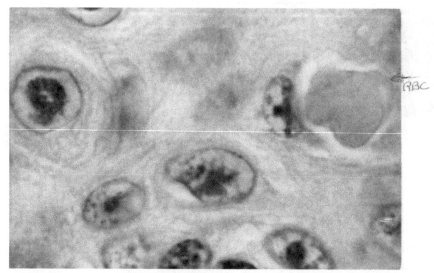

Squamous carcinoma of the lip. Notice in the upper right corner, one of the cancer cells has an RBC within the cytoplasm. Erythrophagocytic activity of cancer cells (engulf RBCs).

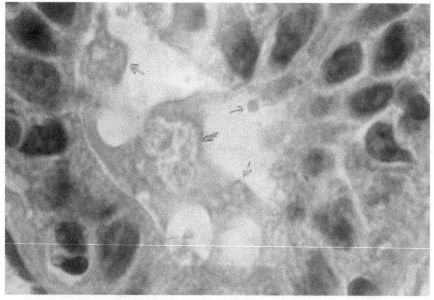

Cancer cells with bacteria in their cytoplasm (Magnification: 10×100)

Cancer Cells Engulf Antibodies. The fact that tumor cells engulf antibodies has been demonstrated with I-131 prelabeled antibodies, and with plasma proteins labeled with radioactive tracers. Babson and Winnick found that the isotope-labeled protein uptake by the tumors was greater than the nontumorous tissue. They labeled plasma with the amino acid leucine or isoleucine with C-14, and administered the radioactive-labeled plasma to tumor-bearing rats. It was noted that the specific activity of the tumor exceeded the protein activity of the liver and the kidneys. Their findings indicated that the tumors (cancers) used the antibodies for its nutrition.

Babson et al. also labeled the plasma with two different amino acids and found that the ratio of the isotopes did not vary in the tumor protein. This points out that the tumor incorporated the whole plasma protein; otherwise, the protein-labeled ratio would have been altered had the proteins been first hydrolized to free amino acids.

They also compared the radioactive B lycine and lysine uptake by the Walker and the Jensen tumors.

Other studies done by Bush and Greene revealed that the uptake of the isotope-labeled free amino acids by the pancreas was much greater than that found in other tissues, and that the actively growing tumor took little amount of the labeled amino acid in vivo compared with the pancreas uptake. However, the tumor uptake of the radioactive plasma proteins was much greater than that of other tissues.

Some tumor cells such as the Ehrlich ascitic cells have a great ability to concentrate amino acids. The amino acid concentration ratio can range from 1.3 to 20.6 of intracellular to extracellular concentration of the amino acids. Bush and Greene noted that the amino acid 2,4-diaminobutyric acid was prominently taken resulting in a noted decrease of the intracellular potassium. However, when tumor-bearing animals were injected with radioactive-labeled amino acids, the uptake by the tumor while exceeding that of the skeletal muscle and kidney could not be compared to the greater amino acid uptake by the liver.

Therefore, the above mentioned experiments demonstrate that the "nitrogen trap" ability of the cancer cells cannot be explained by the ability of the tumors to take or concentrate amino acids, but by the engulfing of the proteins as such.

The preceding findings support my observation that cancer as a parasite nourishes from the readily available protein material in the blood, including antibodies and antibody-coated red blood cells, and it does not necessarily nourishes on amino acids. Cancer thrives off the surrounding proteinmaterial available, manufactured by the healthy lymphoid tissue as an immune response to the cancer-secreted antigens (cancer wastes).

Because of the reduction in the number of efficient mitochondria, cancer cells have a fermentative metabolism which is totally inadequate for normal cell functions. Therefore, the cancer cells' total energy is channeled toward continuous replication as the only means of getting rid of its wastes. The cancer cells have a large nucleus and a scanty cytoplasm. If the cell's organelles are present in the cytoplasm, how can a cancer cell manufacture by itself the necessary nutrients for its survival and for its continuous replication? It has a necessity to be provided by the host's healthy tissues.

Protein and Amino Acid Metabolism. In 1954, Midler et al. concluded that part of the nitrogen contained in a tumor was probably derived from the host's body. He arrived at this conclusion after working with the Walker carcinoma 256, and finding that the nitrogen content of the tumor was greater than the amount of nitrogen stored by the host during the tumor growth. Their findings indicate that the cancerous rats facilitate the breaking down of normal protoplasm, thus providing building blocks for neoplastic tissue growth.

Babson and Winnih in 1954 showed view findings that incompletely hydrolized protein is transferred from healthy tissue to the tissue of the Walker-carcinoma rats. Other experiments showed that the tumor can grow even if the host animal diet was deprived of protein. Radio-labeled amino acid studies have provided evidence that, predominantly, the passage of protein from the host to the tumor is one way. This research supports the view that the tumor's need for protein takes first priority even in a protein-deficient diet.

Reports on nitrogen metabolism in cancer patients vary from positive to a negative balance. In cancer patients, during tumor growth, there is alteration of the amino acids of the blood and tissues, probably related to the cancer and not due to the protein intake.

Korngold and Pressman reported that the Murphy-Sturm lymphosarcoma concentrated antibodies to this tumor. Other researchers, such as LePage, have indicated the apparent preference by neoplastic cells for preformed purines and pyrimidines from outside sources when available. These findings have been verified by Pasieka, who found that both malignant and normal cell lines reduce the glutamine concentration in the medium, but the reduction was greater in the malignant lines.

Pasieka suggested that, perhaps, the normal cell lines had utilized the glutamine because they had already undergone malignant transformation.

Cancer Cells Produce Antigenic Substances. One of the antigenic substances produced by cancer cells is the carcinoembryonic antigen (CEA). Although elevated levels may be identified in noncancerous diseases, such as benign tumors, tuberculosis, pancreatitis, cirrhosis of the liver, inflammatory conditions of the bowel and emphysema, the levels in these conditions are not significantly elevated as in cases of colon and rectal carcinoma metastatic to the liver or bone where the CEA levels of 20mcg or greater may be found.

CEA determinations are useful for evaluation of metastases in cancers of the rectum and colon, and for monitoring therapeutic results. CEA and alphafetoprotein (AFP) are not only produced by cancer cells, but by fetal tissue as well.

Tissue polypeptide antigen (TPA) is secreted into the blood and urine by rapid growing tissues, such as fetal tissues and tumors. Several tumor antigens have been detected and perhaps many more are to be discovered.

Gold and Freeman in 1965 described CEA. At a neutral pH and by electron microscopy, CEA appears as a characteristic twisted rod-shaped particle measuring about $9 \times 40_{nm}$. CEA is a glycoprotein, of which 45 to 57 percent is carbohydrate, and 30 to 46 percent is protein. Egan et al. found that the "N-acetylneuraminic acid is substituted on position 3 of galactose, and that a large portion of the fucose residues must be linked to N-acetylglucosamine." It is interesting to note the likeness between the compositions of the CEA, the blood groups, and subgroups antigens.

In 1972, Davidsohn noted the absence of isoantigens A, B, and H in cancer tissue. The loss of tissue antigen was more significant as the cancer advanced from in situ to invasive and further with metastases. These findings were interpreted as an immunologic dedifferentiation similarly to tissue anaplasia. The cancer tissue antigens were returning to an embryonic behavior.

There is some cross-reactivity between CEA and blood group A substances. Simon and Pearlman proposed that CEAs were not fully developed blood group substances of the ABO system.

There is an abundance of precursor blood group carbohydrates in erythrocytes of fetuses and newborn. This may represent a greater reactivity of fetal or newborn erythrocytes to an antibody against the precursor N-acetylglucosamynil B'—3 galactosyl B'—4 *glycosylceramide*, than to adult RBCs, as reported by Sterns. During wound healing, there is a loss of the AHB antigenic substances. A correlation exists between the growth and the surface properties of cells.

Blood groups' specificity is also found in bacteria. As cancer cells dedifferentiate into a more primitive anaplastic tumor cells, it loses its ability to produce specific blood antigens. Decrease of the ABH antigens has also been observed in leukemia.

The primitive macrophage is the only totipotential cell able of transforming into any tissue as the need arises, not only as a repair mechanism in normal response, but also the macrophage is able to transform into cancer cells under the proper triggering mechanism. On examining sections of cancer tissue, I have observed progressive reactivity and changes of the macrophages at the periphery and within the connective tissue of tumors. There is gradual pleomorphism of the macrophages (connective tissue cells). All the changes observed are characteristic of malignant transformation.

There is some sharing of complementary antigens between the animal and the plant kingdoms since some plant lectins agglutinate RBCs.

Certain beans produce substances called lectins that agglutinate specific red blood cell types within the ABO system. For example, Anti-A1 Dolichous biflorus, Ulex europeus, and Anti-B Sophora japonica are plant lectins that agglutinate RBCs. Dolichous agglutinates RBCs from group A blood, and the Sophora agglutinates group B blood cells.

Cancers secrete various antigenic substances. Carcinoma of the lung, small cell type, has four surface antigens as reported by Robins and Contran. Since these antigens were previously recognized as macrophage surface antigens, Robins et al. concluded that "cancerous cells may arise from macrophages precursors in the bone marrow." As part of the reticuloendothelial system (RES), their findings support our concept of the important role that macrophages play in cancer pathogenesis, and in cancer metastases by in situ transformation of cancer-antigen-primed macrophages (RES).

The cancer antigens form immunocomplexes that coat the cell tissue surfaces including the RBCs. These immunocomplexes and cancer-free antigens are engulfed by the scavenger macrophages. However, with the progressive cancer growth, there is a parallel increase of cancer-antigen (cancer wastes) production. This results in further macrophage sensitization by the cancer-antigen and in situ transformation of macrophages once they have reached their final number of division. Excess immunocomplexes not engulfed by the macrophages, not only coat the cells producing aggregates with the RBCs, but clog the capillaries and are deposited in the interstitial tissue in the form of amyloid. This is a frequent finding in tissue of cancer patients as noted by Dietz and also by Lesher, Grahn, and Sallese. Amyloid deposits and immunocomplexes interfere with the normal tissue physiology by impeding nutritional intake and wastes elimination.

Fibrosarcomas have their characteristic-specific antigens. Korngold and Pressman noted that it was not only necessary to remove the entire tumor, but also to wait for a week after the removal of the tumor, to allow for the disappearance of the antigen prior the test for antigenicity. They also noted that secondary tumors could be induced if the animal was challenged with a fragment of tumor transplant while carrying the primary tumor.

A group of researchers at Wistar produced a monoclonal antibody that reacts and identifies a colorectal cell antigen. The glycolipids produced by the cancer are present on fetal cells, but not in adult cells. This antigen is shed into the blood of the cancer patients. Probably, many other specific antigens are also produced, but yet unknown.

Monoclonal antibodies are being used for cancer diagnosis, localization of cancer, and for cancer therapy. Some patients with leukemia or lymphoma have been treated with monoclonal antibodies and have shown some initial improvement, but eventually the tumor growth progressed rapidly.

It is doubtful that monoclonal therapy will be effective since each type of cell produce specific antigen/s, and all cancers have heterogeneous cell population.

All matters are in constant motion, and the motion or vibration of proteins at the antigenic site depends on many variables such as the pH, temperature, molecular structure, and others. The vibration can be identified by nuclear magnetic resonance (NMR). Each type of atom has a characteristic magnetic field that is modified by the magnetic field of nearby atoms. Therefore, by comparing magnetic fields, alterations are detected and tumors can be identified.

Because alteration of matter can affect vibratory rates with subsequent structural arrangement, it is frightening to think of the consequences of genetic engineering and the possibility of accidental environmental contamination by an unbalanced gene or enzyme. The result can be catastrophic.

Carcinoembryonic Antigen. What makes the cancer cell unrecognizable by the tissue immune system (T lymphocytes)? Do some of the cancer-produced antigens coat the T lymphocytes (thymus-derived), neutralizing it and thus making them nonreactive to the cancerous growth?

The importance of T cells in tissue rejection and control of viral infections is well recognized.

In 1975, Strelkauskas, Wilson, and Dray reported changes to the T and B cell levels in early pregnancy. They suggested that this inversion may be due to a physiological depletion of the suppressor T cells, and that the increased number of B cells observed in the first trimester permitted the allograph uptake by the production of antibodies. This correlates with the decrease in cell-mediated immunity noted in pregnancy. Because of the rise and fall of the T and B cells, it appears to be parallel or a similar variation of the serum human gonadotropin (hCG) levels. Strelkauskas et al. speculated on the possible immunoregulatory effect of hCG. This hormone has been considered responsible for the maternal immunosupression of the fetal tissue and of the immunosupression of the cancer host. Human chorionic gonadotropin has been demonstrated in the cytoplasm and on the surface of malignant cells.

Gold and Freedman described carcinoembryonic antigen in 1965. The antigen determinant of the CEA is located in the protein component.

It has been found that the CEA concentration is higher in cancer than in healthy repair tissue, not only because of the immaturity of the cancer cell, but also due to its rapid growth.

The distribution of the CEA activity may be specific. Evidence has been reported that the CEA antigen is present in tissues infiltrated by macrophages, such as the lung and spleen, also the CEA is found in the gastrointestinal tract. Is it possible that CEA is produced by rapidly growing macrophages as found in healing wounds, traumatized areas with tissue-repair activity, and in cancerous tissues?

Noto and associates, studying 272 pregnant women, reported that a peak level of hCG urinary excretion occurs between the sixtieth and the seventieth day following the onset of the last menstrual period with a titer of about 1:64. There's a gradual decrease in titer in the second and third trimester. A titer higher than 1:64 during the first trimester may indicate hydatiform mole, choriocarcinoma, or other abnormality. Bradbury, Goplerud, McCarthy, and Pennington found elevated levels of hCG in the third trimester of women immunized to anti-Rh, and in those women whose newborn had fetal hydrops.

It has been reported that HCG inhibits the T lymohocytes. This could explain why the fetus is not rejected. Circulating immunocomplexes are present in all normal pregnancies. The immunecomplexes coating the cell membrane could inhibit recognition, and thus, immunetolerance to the fetus could also occur.

In cancer, there are circulating immunecomplexes or blocking factors that inhibit cell immunity. The cancer-antigen combined with the plasma-cell-produced antibodies form complexes. The cancer-antigen and the immunecomplexes, by coating the cells' surfaces, including the RBCs, interfere with the normal cellular metabolism. Cellular wastes are retained with subsequent tissue toxicity and hypoxia. This explains the general fatigue, weakness, cold sensation, malnourishment, and pain as common complains in cancer patients. All of the above, together with the lack of nutrition due to anorexia, and the previously noted erythrophagocytic activity (engulf RBCs) of cancer cells, explain not only the weight loss, but the anemia observed in nonbleeding cancer patients.

With plenty of available nutrients (antibodies and RBCs), cancer cells not only continue to thrive and to replicate endlessly, but also continue to spread by in situ transformation of macrophages.

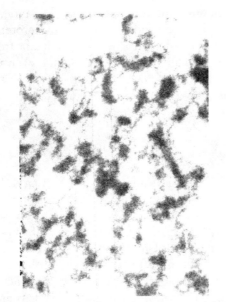

Electron photograph from the plasma globulin of a patient with cancer. Notice the great amount of immunecomplexes present. (Magnification: 8,300)

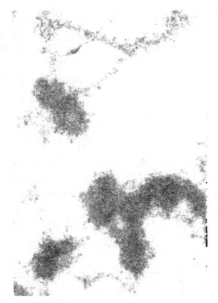

Electron photograph
Same plasma-globulin fraction with greater magnification of the immune complexes (Magnification: 21,000)

Thus, the continuous antibody production, demanded by the stimulus of the cancer antigen, utilizes the body's nutrients and protein material available to the host. This, combined with the usual anorexia frequently present in cancer patients, will gradually produce anemia and eventually cachexia.

Because of the ability of cancer to produce antigens that stimulate the production of antibodies by the plasma cells, cancer then behaves as an autoimmune disease.

Alphafetoprotein

Alfa-fetoprotein (AFP) is produced by the human embryo liver, and it can be detected as early as twenty-nine days after conception. The concentration of AFP increases rapidly from 67 µg/ml at about six and a half weeks of gestation to about 2,000 µg/mL at nine and a half weeks. AFP reaches its peak at ten to thirteen weeks of gestation, with values of approximately 3,000 µg/ml as reported by Gitlin. After the seventeenth week of gestation, the AFP decreases gradually to levels ranging from 13 to 86 µg/mL at term.

The presence of AFP continues to be reduced to around 1 to 2 ng by two years of age. This level is maintained throughout adulthood. The level is highest during the third trimester of pregnancy, when concentrations of up to 500 ng/ml has been reported.

In trophoblastic hyperplasia and in hyditiform mole, there is a production of human chorionic gonadotrophic hormone (HCG). The level indicates the degree of proliferation.

Other organs also synthesize AFP, but to a lesser degree than the liver.

Is the AFP inhibiting the mother's cells from recognizing the fetus as a foreign body and thus incapacitating the host's T cells (T lymphocytes) to react accordingly? Is something similar occurring in cancer, whereby the cancer-antigen-coated cells are inhibited from reacting?

In the first instance, pregnancy is a normal process. But in the case of a mole, like in cancer, both are abnormal processes; yet the body does not reject it.

It is known that parasites can develop in an immune-competent host if they are not recognized as foreign. This can be accomplished if the parasite has the ability to produce molecular mimicry or antigen sharing or to secrete substances that suppress the host's immune system. If this happens with parasites, why not with cancer that behaves as a parasite?

Cancer Cell Plasma Membrane

Cancer Cell Plasma Membrane. The cancer cell plasma membrane plays a fundamental part in cancer immunebiology. It is at this level where the secretion of the cancer antigen/s takes place.

When in high concentration, antigens secreted by the cancer cells have an inhibitory activity against the immune lymphocytes. These cancer antigens sensitize the lymphocytes to the engulfing activity of the macrophages, and thus, the lymphocytes are destroyed.

Examination of lymph nodes with Hodgkin's disease showed most of the lymphocytes opposed to neoplastic cells to be positive for acid phosphatase activity within their Golgi zone. This acid phosphatase activity is characteristic of the thymus-dependent (T) lymphocytes. Studies of direct immunology demonstrate the apposed lymphocytes in Hodgkin's disease to be T lymphocytes, but the immunoglobulin-positive non–T cells to be the neoplastic Reed-Sternberg cells.

In vivo phagocytosis by macrophages of Hodgkin's antigen-coated T cells have been demonstrated by electron microscopy.

While T lymphocytes can be stimulated by low concentrations of tumor antigens, higher concentrations have the opposite effect: it inhibits the T cells' activity. However, the plant mitogen phytohemagglutinin (PHA; stimulates mitosis, cell division), selectively marked for T lymphocytes, reactivates the T lymphocytes. In addition to the tumor-antigen binding sites, the T lymphocytes plasma membrane has PHA binding sites.

Tumor-antigen-coated T cells are identified by the macrophages as tumor cells, and are engulfed as the engulfed tumor-antigen-coated RBC, as demonstrated in my studies of cancer tissues.

By the very action of assimilating the tumor antigen and cancer cell wastes, the macrophage (RES) became primed by it, and eventually transformed in situ into cancer cells once it has reached the limited number of normal division.

Heterogeneity of Cancer Cells. It is a known fact that the regeneration of whole plants from fragments of mature organs is possible. There is strong supporting evidence that "plant cells retain genetic totipotency through differentiation" as noted by Osborne. Although within the intact plant, there are intrinsic controls that maintain a normal pattern of growth. For example, the genes responsible for the manifestation of the petal color must be carried in all flowering plant cells, although normally their expression is repressed.

There is increasing evidence that almost all, if not all, cancers have a diverse and heterogeneous cellular morphology. This is manifested not only by morphological variations, but also by variations in hormone receptors, expression of membrane-surface antigens, ability to spread, karyotype, and several other characteristics. Also, clonogenic cell have a great capacity for manifesting stem cell properties and heterogeneity. Buick and Pollack have concluded that "control of cell proliferation and differentiation in renewing tissues depend on both control of cell cycle entry and on the probability of stem cell renewal."

Morphologic Versatility of Cancer Cells

Experimentally and clinically, the morphologic versatility of cancer cells and its variations in metastases have been demonstrated.

Although probably high, the exact number of phenotypically specific tumor cells' subpopulation in various tumors is unknown. Cancerous tumors in different stages of development may show an infinite variety of cellular population and phenotype variations.

At a point, cellular variations may be the result of what the primitive macrophage may have been primed (by engulfing cancer cells fragments and wastes). The macrophages, being scavengers, are very active if provoked by body wastes or by injury. With the continuous production of wastes by the cancer, there will be active replication of macrophages in order to keep up with the growing accumulation of cancer wastes or antigenic substances.

However, when the macrophages reach the critical number of division, it will transform into cancer cell since it has been primed by the cancer waste.

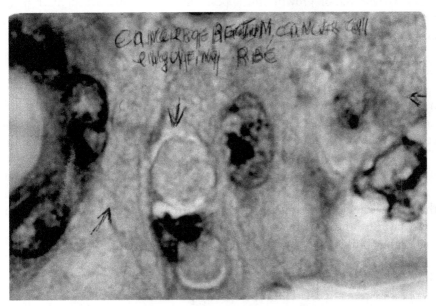

Rectal tissue showing cell transformation in close proximity to cancer of the rectum (Magnification: 10×100)

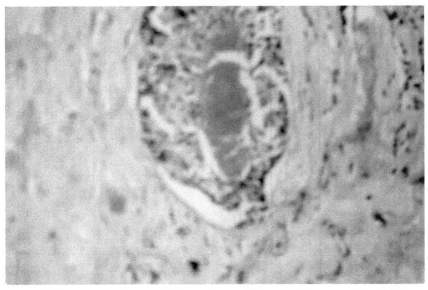

Infiltrating mucus-producing adenocarcinoma of rectum. Notice pleomorphysm of cancer cells. (Magnification: 10×100)

This new tumor growth will appear where the transformed macrophages happen to be—lymph nodes, liver, lung, and others; thus, metastases predominantly occur.

The transformed macrophage then behaves as a cancer cell and not as a normal macrophage, although it still maintains its phagocytic activity.

Fidler and Kripke investigated the potential ability of the primary tumor to metastasize by injecting intravenously saline suspension of tumor cells and by doing evaluation for pulmonary metastases. Part of the saline-suspended tumor cells were cloned, isolated, and tested experimentally for their metastatic ability. The uncloned and cloned sublines would have the same number of metastases if the original tumor cells contained metastatic potential. But according to the researchers, the result proved this not to be the case. They observed that while the original uncloned parental tumor cells' group produced the same number of metastases in different animals, the cloned sublines varied widely in their metastatic ability.

Their findings demonstrated the heterogeneity of the primary tumor, since control of subcloning experiments demonstrated that the variations in metastases were not related to the cloning process.

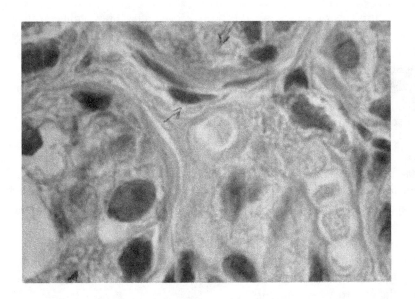

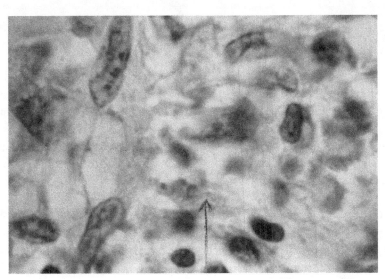

Transformation of macrophages in areas adjacent to cancerous tissue
Adenocarcinoma of rectum with nearby transforming macrophages

Macrophages Precursors as Totipotential Cells

Mature macrophages are the body scavengers. They collect cell wastes or any particulate foreign matter within the body, including cholesterol. Focal aggregates of cholesterol-laden macrophages are frequently seen in arteriosclerotic plaques.

Macrophages precursors are totipotential cells capable of transforming, when need be, into repair tissue, new capillaries, scars, and others. They are indispensable for the body repair.

Under the proper stimulus, by specific antigens, the macrophages precursors may be able to transform into different cells with various morphologic characteristics. Traber et al. have reported that monocytes in culture are transformed into macrophages. Could it be that the macrophages do not derive from the monocytes as Traber et al. concluded, but instead that the monocytes are derived from the macrophages?

Since macrophages are totipotential cells, and more primitive than the monocytes, when monocytes in culture are transformed into macrophages, are they not reverting to a more primitive scavenger form in order to adapt to an artificial in vitro environment?

The Macrophage, (RES): Our Lives' Clock

Connective tissue cells, fibroblasts, endothelial cells, basal cells, regenerative cells, and primitive bone marrow cells are all derived from undifferentiated macrophage, and all are part of the reticuloendothelial system (RES). These cells can participate in the tissue repair or act as scavengers. It is during the scavenger function when these cells become sensitized by the appropriate antigen, and develop into plasma cells and/or metastases according to the age or number of divisions that the cell has gone through. It is evident that the macrophages are essential. But what does all of this has to do with life span?

All normal cells, including macrophages, have a limited life span. But if the life span of a cell depends on a specific number of cell divisions, then the more often cells divide, the sooner they will reach the fiftieth division. At this point, the cells either die or transform.

Macrophages divide more frequently than any other cell in the body.

Functioning as primordial blood cells.

Acting as scavengers, and first line of defense against bacteria, viruses, or any particulate matter.

They divide to foreign storage bodies and adipose tissue.

36

It has been demonstrated that when the life span of fibroblasts (macrophages) reaches up to the fiftieth division, one of two things happen: either the cells die or they transform. This indicates that the more the macrophages are provoked into dividing, the sooner they will reach the end of their life span. The stimulus for division can be the result of injuries and diseases. All these conditions occurring during fetal life may shorten the life span and/or predispose the newborn to diseases in early life, thus shortening the life span of the newborn if diseases occur in uterus. This could explain why serious diseases such as neuroblastomas and leukemia may appear early in life.

After the fiftieth division, when the cell reaches old age, the cell is then a candidate for cell transformation since its oxidative functions are impaired, and it is more susceptible to be transformed if it has the oncogene, and/or it is infected by an appropriate oncogenic virus.

If the patient does not have oncogenes, then when the cells reach their fiftieth division, there will be a progressive rapid decline of the individual's health with aging and degenerative diseases, since the repair mechanism represented by the macrophages has been exhausted. The life's time clock has ran out.

Cancer Cell Nucleus

In the cancer cell, the nucleus is where the genetic material is contained within the chromosomes. Cancer cells have large nucleocytoplasmic ratio. The scanty cytoplasm does not have enough space to accommodate the necessary organelles in adequate amounts to be able to manufacture the required nutrients as normal cells do. In normal cells, the greater part of the cell is represented by the cytoplasm where the numerous metabolic activities are performed. However, in the cancer cell, the opposite occurs.

In the cancer cell, the nucleus represents most of the cell while the cytoplasm is reduced to a perinuclear halo.

Because of the limited number of organelles in a cancer cell, the nutrients have to be readily available and be manufactured outside the cancer cell itself. The cancer cell's fermentative metabolism reverts to a primitive cell physiology. With its basic physiology, a cancer cell survives by being scavenger. It lives off the antibody-coated RBCs and plasma antibodies. The plasma membrane of cancer cell is more electropositive than the membrane of a normal cell. This electropositivity of the cancer cell attracts electronegative molecules such as antibodies.

The cancer cell nuclear membrane is thicker and more prominent than the nuclear membrane of a normal cell. It also shows gaps or spaces between the membrane and the nucleus.

The nucleus is not only larger, but more darkly stained, more basophilic, very pleomorphic, anaplastic, and frequently in mitosis (cell division). The mitotic activity is also morphologically abnormal. There is variation in appearance and number of the chromosomes, and changes are observed from one clone to the next clone of cancer cells.

The cancer cell nucleus has lost its normal control. With all the nuclear alterations, it is easy to understand the pleomorphism of cancer cells and its variation potential.

During normal cell division, the like chromosomes pair and replicate each other. However, in cancer, there is a chaotic composition of chromosomes; and the normal pairing cannot occur. What initiates the drastic changes that transform a normal cell into a cancer cell? Is there a virus-cell integration triggering the changes?

Cancer Cell Ribosomes. Abiditsch-Mays and Breitfellner, based on electron microscope observations, reported that "ribosomes not only those of the endoplasmic reticulum, but also free ribosomes are very rare" in cancer cells. Ribosomes are the cell's organelles essential to the cell's normal functions and for manufacturing substances as commanded by the nucleus in response to the cell's needs.

In normal cells, the messenger RNA (mRNA) interacts with ribosomes to form polyribosomes, and it is on these polyribosomes where protein synthesis occurs. Having marked reduction on the number of ribosomes, cancer cells are unable to perform this function.

Acidic pH of Cancer Cell. Oxygen is harmful to cancer cells. Cancer cells thrive in an anaerobic environment. Since an acidic medium facilitates the release of oxygen, it is easy to understand why cancer cells have an acidic pH of 6.8. The acid pH of cancer cells may also explain why cancer cells have a preference for calcium, since calcium deposits are in acidic medium.

Every living organism must be able to get rid of its waste products in order to survive; the cancer cell is not an exception. Because of its rapid metabolism and growth, it must produce more wastes than the average normal cell. However, the cancer cell plasma membrane is more rigid and less permeable than that of the normal cell. Due to the rigidity of the cancer cell membrane (just like the shell of an egg or the membranes of an embryo sac), it may not be able to easily eliminate its metabolites through it; and therefore, the cancer cell has to resort to cell division in order to get rid not only of its wastes, but also of the excess unpaired DNA, RNA, and protein material engulfed by the cancer cell. Therefore, there is no end to the cancer cell reproductive cycle.

The waste products of the cancer cell are composed of urea and aldehydes with minute amounts of formaldehyde, among other things. Because of the cancer cell's fermentative metabolism and poor mitochondria function, it cannot oxidize and neutralize its wastes; these wastes act as stimulus for cell division. Formaldehyde, one of the cancer cell's wastes, is a known carcinogenic and a promoter of cell division. Retention of minute amounts of formaldehyde promotes continuous cancer cell division.

Formaldehyde hardens proteins and makes them insoluble. For this reason, it is used in the laboratory to fix, harden, and preserve tissues. The presence of formaldehyde, in combination with calcium, in an infinitesimal amount in the cancer cell as a waste product may be responsible for the rigidity of the cancer cell's plasma membrane.

Chapter II

Cancer as an Immune Disease

Babson and Winnick demonstrated the avidity of cancer cells for proteins, but not particularly for amino acids. Since antibodies are proteins, the antibody production of plasma cells, under the stimulus of the cancer antigen, may end contributing to the cancer nutrition and growth. Humoral antibodies have no effect in cancerous tissue rejection.

Since it has been demonstrated that cancer cells trap antibodies, why not engulf the readily available antibodies (food) produced by the plasma cells as the result of the cancer-antigen stimulus?

Are the plasma cells so overtaxed by the cancer-specific antigen that they are unresponsive to any other antigenic stimulus? Thus, cancer patients, particularly at the end stage of the disease, become anergic (unresponsive) and therefore susceptible to bacterial, fungal, and viral infections.

Are the plasma cells nonresponsive because their antigenic sites are obliterated or blocked off by the cancer antigen and by immune complexes to the point that there are no antigenic sites available for any other type of immune response, but only to the cancer stimulus?

This will make the cancer patient more susceptible to infections regardless of the amount of the immunoglobulin present in the cancer patient's plasma since all of the immunoglobulin produced by the plasma cells is cancer-specific antigen, and therefore, it will not protect the patient against infections. With the plasma cell's antigenic sites saturated with the cancer antigen, there will be no antigenic site in the plasma cells that will be able to respond to any other antigenic stimulus.

Thus, the continuous antibody-production demand by the cancer antigen utilizes the body's nutrients and proteinaceous material available to the host.

This, together with the usual anorexia present in cancer patients, will gradually produce anemia, general weakness, and eventually caquexia.

Because of the ability of cancer to produce antigens that stimulate the production of antibodies by plasma cells, cancer behaves as an autoimmune disease in effect.

The cancer antigen, combined with the plasma-cell-produced antibodies, form immunocomplexes. With the coating of the immune cells and all tissue cells, including the RBCs, the normal cellular processes are inhibited or slowed down. The antibodies-coated cells cannot exchange nutrients and/or oxygen with its environment. Consequently, cellular wastes are retained, and there will be tissue toxicity and hypoxia.

With plenty of available nutrients (antibodies and RBCs), cancer cells not only continue to thrive and to replicate endlessly, but also spread in the form of in situ transformation of the cancer-primed macrophages (RES).

Initiation of Cancer. How is cancer initiated? Whoever answers this question may unlock the knowledge to life itself. Does cancer growth depend on a single or multiple factors for its development? The present consensus of opinion is that there are multiple factors influencing the occurrence of cancer. There is evidence to support a genetic component in the occurrence of some cancers.

One of the oncology concepts is that cancer cells can express fetal structural genes for specific enzymes and also antigenic proteins, such as the alphafetoprotein and the carcinoembryonic antigen.

Other factors, such as sensitizers and promoters, play a central part in the incidence of cancer. For example, subcutaneously embedded plastic material in rodents induces formation of fibrous pockets with 30–40 percent of tumor incidence. It has been demonstrated, by microscopic examination, the variation in rates of the fibroblastic proliferation in relation with the nature of the plastic used. It was found that the incidence of tumor depended not only in the kind of plastic used, but also in the length of time that the implant was left in place. Examination of the tumors showed variation in cells from hyperplasia, dysplasia, and carcinoma in situ to infiltrating and metastasizing carcinoma. This full spectrum of changes gives an idea of how cancer progresses, and how it can appear in one site or be multifocal.

Is cancer virus dependent? If so, why are viruses so infrequently associated or not found in cancer tissue especially human cancers? Are the viruses so integrated with the cell's organelles that no recognizable viral particles are produced by the host's viral-infected cells?

When human cells in culture were infected with the Simian virus 40 (SV40), the cells proliferated into various stages. Some cells underwent lysis, others proliferated, and the surviving transformed cells, although apparently free of infectious virus, were capable of indefinite proliferation as Hayflick reported.

Does cancer initiation depend on the haploid mating of a specific viral circular DNA with the mitochondrial circular DNA? Does this mating change the physiology of the mitochondria from the normal cell aerobic or oxidative metabolism to an anaerobic or fermentative metabolism, the cancer cell metabolism?

Is cancer initiated or triggered only when compatible viral circular DNA infests or mates with the circular DNA of the mitochondria in a genetically cancer-predisposed cell?

Once the mating occurs between the circular DNA of the proper virus and the circular DNA of the mitochondria, the virus could become integrated with the cellular structure and thus unidentifiable.

Since the DNA of both the mitochondria and the virus are tightly coiled, it must uncoil prior to mating or pairing for the final integration to occur. Once the integration occurs, its stability may be insured by disulfide bonds (R-S-S-R) between two amino acids such as occurs in the amino acid cystine.

What are the events taking place after this integration? Does the virus-mitochondria-integrated circular DNA take over the cell metabolism and control from the nuclear DNA?

The configuration of proteins depends on the pH of the medium. A change in pH can induce electrostatic interactions resulting in changes in the stereoscopic configuration of the protein and in modifications in the enzymatic activity of one or more enzymes. This alteration may support the initiation and/or continuation of the cancer metabolism.

It is a known fact that enzymes need, among other things, an optimal pH for effective function. The integration of extra nucleic acids and proteins from a viral origin into the mitochondria could reduce the intracellular pH to a more acidic medium, thus inhibiting normal enzymes, and at the same time producing other enzymes that favor the cancer metabolism. Therefore, the cell's steady state is altered. Consequently, instead of a normal oxidative metabolism, there is a fermentative metabolism—the cancer metabolism.

Let's assume that mitochondria DNA becomes impregnated with the genetic complementary oncogenic virus; and thus, as a metabolite, a "fetal antigen" is produced by the infected cell. This "fetal antigen" could inhibit or suppress the T cells from reacting to the mitochondria-virus integration.

As other antigenic substances are produced by the transformed, now-cancer cell, the plasma cells will be stimulated to produce antibodies which in turn will be utilized as nutrients by cancer. Mitochondria susceptibility to viral impregnation depends on the cell age. Only cells that have reached their fiftieth division are susceptible to be infected by a complementary oncogenic virus. Once infected, the cell metabolism changes from oxidative to fermentative.

The poorly developed mitochondria of transformed cells will not be able to produce oxidative enzymes, and there will also be a reduction or lack of ATP production.

My hypothesis is: in a genetically cancer-prone individual, when certain aging cells reach their fiftieth division, it alters its metabolism to a plantlike physiology, thus becoming receptive to be impregnated by an oncogenic virus. Once the proper oncogenic virus attacks the aging cell, the impregnation will occur only if the viral circular DNA is complementary to the aging cell mitochondria circular DNA. Once the mitochondrial DNA impregnation by the viral DNA takes place, fetal antigen is produced.

The fetal antigen inhibits the T cells from reacting to it, thus rejection of the newly developed cancer cells does not occur. Other antigenic substances are produced by the cancer and these act on the B cells (bursa-derived), plasma cells produce cell to react and produce antibodies. But B cells antibodies are humoral in nature and are not directly tissue antibodies; therefore, it will not have any damaging effect upon the cancer cells. On the contrary, as previously noted, the antibodies will be engulfed by the cancer cells and utilized it as ready-made nutrients. Thus, after the mitochondrion-virus impregnation, the mitochondrion takes over the cellular control from the nucleus. An endless cellular division cycle had started.

Pathobiology of Cancer Cells. Normal cell mitochondria will produce ATP H_2O, CO_2, infinitesimal amounts of formaldehyde, and a superoxide ozone (O_3). Cancer cells impaired mitochondria do not produce O_3 that in normal cells will neutralize the formaldehyde oxidizing it to form a less offensive acid such as formic acid. In cancer cells, due to ineffective mitochondria, no ozone is produced. There is no neutralization of the formaldehyde which is then retained in the cancer cell, and which will drive it to endless division.

The presence of the formaldehyde being a polymerizer will also affect the nuclear DNA resulting in subsequent alterations and pleomorphism of the chromosomes.

In normal cells, the formic acid, together with ammonia, will create amino acids, but since no ozone is produced in cancer cells, the formaldehyde cannot be neutralized to formic acid. But the cancer cell produces sulfur (SH_2) instead of ozone (O_3). The sulfur will be transformed into sulfuric acid (S_4H_2), by SH_2 + H_2O (water). The sulfuric acid in the cancer cells will produce heat and burning sensations. It will increase the rate of molecular vibrations and instability.

In the normal cell, the ozone produced neutralizes the formaldehyde, and the normal cycle continues. But in cancer cells, ozone is not produced; and hence, formaldehyde is not neutralized.

Cancer as a Microscopic Embryo. Each cancer cell does behave as a microscopic embryo. The endogenous part of this embryo is provided by a genetically predisposed aged cell. The cancer genetic predisposition may be located in the mitochondria circular DNA and/or the nuclear DNA. The exogenous part (sperm) of the cancer embryo, do arrive via the oncogenic virus and/or environmental elements. Cancer promoters and/or sensitizers, such as certain chemicals or radiation, stimulate the cancer promoters and activate the cancer tendency.

It is necessary for the oncogenic virus circular DNA to match or be complementary to the genetically cancer-prone-mit circular DNA. Both circular DNAs have to match like "lock and key." If the match is perfect, then the seed for cancer has been planted. The proper match is indispensable; otherwise, the incidence of cancer would be much greater.

Leonard Hayflick and others, by culturing fibroblasts, have demonstrated that about the fiftieth division, the fibroblasts die or are transformed into immortal cells with the capacity to replicate endlessly. Normal cells have a limited number of divisions and therefore a limited life span.

Aged cells, the ones that have reached the fiftieth division, are the ones susceptible to be impregnated by the proper virus in cancer-predisposed individuals. It is then that the complementary virus circular DNA has to join with its corresponding mitochondrial circular DNA.

Tadaro, Green, and Swift reported on the susceptibility of human diploid fibroblast strains to transform in culture by oncogenic virus (SV40). They noted that cells from patients with Fanconi's anemia (an autosomal disease associated with high incidence of chromosome anomalies and tumors) resulted ten times higher incidence of cell transformation.

Cancer Cell, the Survival of the Fittest. Are cancer cells the survival of the fittest? Are normal cells transformed into cancer cells when they are old, and when the pollution of the cellular environment is such that the cells will die if they did not have the ability to transform into cancer scavenger cells?

Can anyone develop cancer, or is there need for a genetic predisposition? Is there a close interplay between the genetic component (predisposition) and the environment? Let's suppose that a person has the gene for cancer of the lung, but he/she does not smoke and does live a healthy life in a clean environment. Will that person develop cancer anyway? On the other hand, can a person with no cancer gene develop cancer if exposed to carcinogenic substances?

Macrophage Role in Cancer Pathogenesis and in Metastases

What part does the macrophage play in cancer pathogenesis? Macrophages are the body scavengers. They are present everywhere in the body, in the blood and any other tissue. Fibroblasts and connective tissue cells are also macrophages. Macrophages are one of the most abundant cells in the body. They also represent the reticuloendothelial system (RES). Macrophages are the cells that help heal wounds, form new blood vessels and scars, engulf foreign particles, such as carbon particles in the lung, or ingest bacteria, fungi, or extravasated RBCs.

Ghadially and Perry, studying the human hepatocellular carcinoma by electron microscopy, found lack of desmosomes and lysosomes. Concurrently, they also noted the significant finding of the absence of endothelial and Kupffer cells lining the sinusoids. Were the reticuloendothelial cells (RES) already transformed into cancer cells and therefore not present as such?

Macrophages are present in the inflammatory infiltrate of cancerous tissue. There are contradictory reports in the literature regarding the inflammatory infiltrate in cancerous tissue. Inflammatory infiltrate is usually composed of lymphocytes, plasma cells, and macrophages. In 1921–1922, William McCarthy was the first to call attention to the favorable effect that chronic inflammatory infiltrate plays in certain cancers, such as cancer of breast, rectum, and stomach. He felt that the chronic inflammatory infiltrate may have a part in the defense mechanism of the body. Similar claims of the beneficial effect to the host from the inflammatory reaction to the cancer have been made in experimental animals.

The protective effect of the inflammatory infiltrate appears to be better in carcinomas than in connective tissue tumors or sarcomas.

Testicular seminoma, medullary carcinoma of breast, and Hodgkin's disease are tumors in which lymphocytes predominate. These malignancies are known to have a better prognosis than other types of tumors involving the same organs. Some reports disclaim the beneficial effect of the inflammatory infiltrate in cancer, although the majority of the published evidence favors its benefits. But in the chronic inflammatory infiltrate, there are several kinds of cells: lymphocytes, plasma cells, and macrophages or histiocytes (RES). Of these cells, which one or ones are responsible for the beneficial effect?

Are the T lymphocytes, the B lymphocytes, the plasma cells, or the macrophages, individually or the combination of all of them, responsible for the benefit?

If the antigen produced by the cancer cells in part inhibits the T cells, and on the other it stimulates the B cells (B lymphocyte) to produce plasma cells, that in turn will produce immunoglobulins, anti-cancer-antigen antibodies. However, this antibody, being humoral in nature, has no damaging effect on the cancer cells.

With the neutralization of the T cells, killer cells, by the fetal-cancer antigen and the stimulation of the B cells by other cancer antigens to produce antibodies, an ideal situation has been created by the cancer for its growth and proliferation, since cancer utilizes antibodies for its nourishment.

The only cell left from the triad of T cells and B cells are the macrophages (the scavengers). When the production of cancer antigen and antibodies are in excess of the amount required for the survival of the cancer cells, the unwanted excess is engulfed by the macrophages. Any leftover antigen, antibody, or immunocomplexes are deposited within the interstitial tissue in the form of amyloid, rich in lipoproteins and mucopolysacharides. Amyloid deposits are frequent findings in cancer connective tissue.

The macrophages, upon engulfing the cancer antigen, become primed and sensitized to the cancer cell's genetic characteristics. Thus, as cancer-primed macrophages divide and are stimulated by the great and inexhaustible amount of cancer antigens, they reach their fiftieth division and are transformed in situ into cancer cells.

Since the sensitized and stimulated primitive or embryonal macrophages are totipotential in their ability to form various tissues, the transformed or metastatic cells, may or may not necessarily resemble the original tumor. This explains the multiclonal and pleomorphic ability of the cancer cells.

Hayflick has stated, "On the basis of the in vitro data, the fibroblast may represent the upper limit of proliferative potential."

Hibbs reported that in vitro, activated macrophages selectively destroy cancer cells while normal cells are not affected. In vivo studies also found that the macrophages tumor resistance is provoked by the various synthetic and biological immunostimulants.

Kaplan and Horohan suggested "that activated macrophages may be present systematically in the immunopotentiator-treated tumor-bearing host." Macrophage participation at the effector level is needed by the sensitized lymphocytes for effective transfer of specific tumor immunity.

While antibodies to the tumor antigens, in the presence of complement, can be cytotoxic to the tumor cells, antitumor antibodies could intensify tumor growth.

Antitumor antibody and antigen have been eluted from patients with malignancy and associated nephrotic syndrome. Lewis et al. suggested that "the presence of these various antibodies or immunocomplexes in malignacy demonstrates a derangement characterized by a breaking of immune regulation, rather than either a total lack of immunity or a 'weak reaction to the so called "weak" tumor antigens'."

The preceding supports my concept of how metastases occur. Macrophages, the body scavengers, on engulfing the cancer antigen/s and immunocomplexes are sensitized. With progression of the disease, there is marked and continuous production of antibodies with oversaturation of the antigenic sites. As multiplication of the macrophages persists, they will eventually reach their transforming point. At this level, in order for the macrophages to survive the patient's polluted environment, and better serve the host, it will transform. It will change its metabolism from a normal oxidative to a pathologic or anaerobic metabolism, a cancer cell metabolism. Therefore, most of the so-called metastases occur by in situ transformation of the cancer antigen primed aged macrophages. This does not exclude the possibility of metastases occurring by aggregates of detached cancer cells traveling through blood vessels or lymphatics, and implanting in other tissues and organs. While this latter way of metastasis could explain metastases in an active primary cancer, it does not explain the recurrence of cancer or metastases in previously operated and treated cases, where there is no trace of remaining cancer, and yet years later metastases occur.

However, in situ transformation of cancer-primed macrophages explains how metastases appear years later after complete recovery from cancer. The cancer-primed macrophages lay dormant in the tissues until months or years later when they are provoked to divide by current emotional upsets and infections, thus reaching their fiftieth division and transforming in situ brain, lung, liver, etc. wherever they happen to be, and so metastases occur.

Each transformed macrophage will divide and produce a clone of malignant cells that may or not resemble the primary cancer. This clone will represent metastases due to the transformation of macrophage in situ. The clone morphology can vary according the maturation level of the macrophages when they were sensitized or primed by the cancer antigen/s.

Therefore, according to my concept, metastases primarily occur by in situ transformation of the tumor-antigen-primed macrophage when it has reached the last number of normal division that a healthy cell can have.

Could it be possible that as tumor cells die, bits of the tumor's genetic materials, acting as jumping genes, infest the macrophages, and so promote further cell transformation?

Amamoto and colleagues reported in Science how to transform fresh human leukocytes by culturing it with irradiated T cell leukemia virus cell lines. They found integration of the primed ATLV genomes into the normal leukocytes. ATLV (adult T cell leukemia) is a retrovirus. Retroviruses use their DNA host for its own transcription. DiBernardino and colleagues noted the reactivation of the erythrocytes genes of Rana, a cold blooded animal, "when transplanted in the cytoplasm of maturing oocytes. to form swimming tadpoles." They concluded that there was reactivation of the dormant RBC genes while conditioning the oocytes' cytoplasm.

When there is a rapidly growing tumor, more cancer antigen and antibodies are being produced; and hence, most likely, the more immature the macrophages are going to be primed. Therefore, the metastases will appear more pleomorphic, and more primitive, or undifferentiated. It will resemble less the primary tumor; it will be more anaplastic.

Dr. Isaiah J. Fidler, Chairman of the Department of Cell Biology at the University of Texas has stated, "that metastases are not produced by the random survival of cells detaching from the primary tumor, but rather, metastases, in general, are produced from selective growth of specialized malignant cells that persist within the parental tumor."

Macrophages, Platelets and Other Growth Factors

Macrophages produce a growth factor that participates in wound healing, in connective tissue formation, and in fibroblastic proliferation. When this activity is inhibited by the local administration of anti-macrophage sera in a monocytopenic animal, the rate of fibroblastic proliferation, connective tissue formation, and wound healing is reduced.

A growth factor from platelets has been extracted in various laboratories. This platelet factor stimulates mitotic activity. Simian sarcoma virus (SSV) transformed normal rat kidney secretes in the culture medium a mitogen similar to platelet-derived growth factor (PDGF).

An endothelial cell-derived growth factor has also been purified. Macrophages are present in all arteriosclerotic changes, and previously, it was stated that there is a growth factor in macrophages. An epidermal-growth factor (EGF) in cell culture stimulates the growth of various cell types.

Heterogeneity of Cells in Malignant Tumors

Variations in the cell morphology within a tumor have been known since last century with the microscopic studies of tumors.

Some tumors are heterogeneous with different subpopulations of tumor cells. Each population of tumor cells may have differences including growth rate, metastatic ability, karyotype, biochemical properties, antigenicity, chemotherapeutic susceptibility, and immunogenicity.

In 1939, Koch et al. worked with the Ehrlich carcinoma and isolated a subline from these tumor cells that metastasize readily. He then suggested that in a particular tumor may be cells with various metastatic capabilities. The various and pleomorphic patterns of maligned tumors and their metastases are common knowledge to *pathologists* (medical doctors specialized in the study of diseases and their tissue manifestations).

Some tumors have a diverse cell population. In 1981, Fidler et al. reported on the phenotype diversity in a murine melanoma of recent origin.

Tumor-Associated Antigens

There are antigens associated with benign and malignant tumors. Antigens are also found in normal tissues, fetal and adult organs included.

It was hoped that these antigens were cancer specific for the use of cancer diagnosis, but since there is a wide distribution of the carcinoembryonic antigen (CEA) in nonmalignant conditions, this test is unreliable unless present in a significantly elevated titer.

When CEA was reported in 1965, it was believed to be specifically associated with embryonic colon and cancer of the gastrointestinal tract in humans.

Subsequently, it found several other cancers, bronchogenic carcinomas and cancer of the breast included. Trace amounts of CEA have been found in normal colon.

Other diseases may show CEA (e.g., uremia, cirrhosis of the liver, diabetes). CEA has been found in patients suffering from artheriosclerosis, chronic obstructive lung disease, collagen disease, and other diseases.

If the CEA-secreting cancer is resected, the CEA level returns to normal, but it will increase the appearance of metastases.

Alphafetoprotein is present in fetal serum and in about 50–80 percent of the sera from patients with primary liver cancer. This alpha-1 globulin is also present in 2 percent of patients with other liver diseases including viral hepatitis.

However, increased levels of alphafetoprotein (AFP) are significant for the diagnosis of cancer of the liver if the patient is not suffering from hepatitis.

Fetal-sulphoglycoprotein antigen (FSA) was demonstrated by immunodiffusion in fetal stomach and in the gastric juice of 96 percent of the patients with histologic diagnosis of carcinoma of the stomach. It also was found in 9 percent of other gastric diseases and in normal people.

Why is there such a variety of growth factors and or antigenic substances in malignant tumors? Is the variety related to the multiplicity of the tumor cellular pattern?

Each variety of primitive cells may produce a specific cellular waste or antigen according to its developmental stage and thus explains not only the heterogeneous appearance of the tumors, but also the variety of cancer-produced antigenic substances.

The type of antigen/s produced by a particular cancer will depend then in the differentiation or undifferentiation of its cellular components.

Sinus Histiocytic Hyperplasia in Lymph Nodes

In literature, hyperplasis of histiocytes (macrophages) in the lymph nodes sinuses have been reported as a sign of good omen or good prognosis for the cancer patient.

In the early stages of tumor growth, there is hyperplasia of the small lymphocytes in lymph nodes, especially in the cortical and paracortical (thymus-dependent) areas. This is detected by the presence of large pyroninophylic (methylgreen pyronine positive) immunoblasts. Their presence is accepted as an indication of the body resistance to the tumor growth. These cells are stimulated lymphocytes and are similar to the cells transformed by phytohemagglutinins.

The further development of the tumor is characterized by follicular cell (B cell) hyperplasia of the lymph nodes and with subsequent appearance of plasma cells.

In the terminal stage of cancer, there is usually a depletion of the lymphoid cell population, but there is some sinus histiocytic proliferation. The presence of follicular hyperplasia (macrophages), alone or associated with plasma cell hyperplasia, signals a poor prognosis.

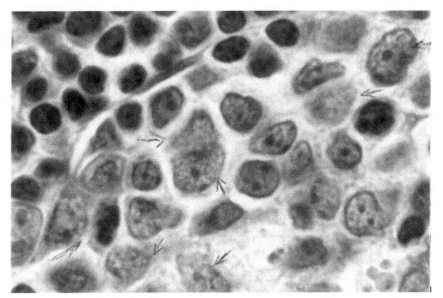

Lymph node from axilla, from a case of carcinoma of breast. Notice reactivity of follicular cells (RES).

Are these cells going to be transformed into cancer cells?

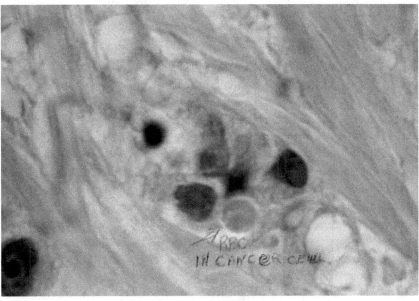

Infiltrating adenocarcinoma of breast (Magnification: 10×100)

It is interesting to note that the immunological response to cancer with production of humoral antibody correlates with the enhancement of tumor growth as demonstrated experimentally in mice by Kalis.

The findings of increased numbers of plasma cells and of sinus histiocytic (macrophages) hyperplasia, associated with the increase of humoral antibodies, signaling a poor prognosis (outcome), supports the concept that cancer thrives on antibodies and on antibodies-coated RBCs. But when the host is so debilitated that it cannot manufacture enough nutrients (antibodies, etc.), then the patient dies.

Vaccination Effect on Cancer

Vaccination stimulates antibody production and tumor growth. However, because sometimes there is a cytotoxic effect, as the result of the vaccine, vaccination has been used to treat cancer patients in association with other therapeutic modalities, such as irradiation, transfusion of lymphocytes, and others, all without much success.

Various results are reported in literature. Some studies indicate that this form of therapy does not produce general immunestimulation, but that it essentially activates the macrophages.

Since cancer thrives on proteins and antibodies, as proven by Babson and Winnick, and vaccination stimulates antibody production, it is easy to understand not only the failures, but also the potential danger of this therapeutic approach.

Inflammatory Infiltrate in Cancer

In 1921–1922, McCarthy associated the chronic inflammatory reaction in cancer "as possible part of the defense mechanism." Thereafter, this subject has been deviated. The favorable effect of the infiltrate refers predominantly to tumors of epithelial origin than sarcomas. A similar beneficial effect has been reported in animals.

Chronic inflammation is characteristic of autografted tumors undergoing rejection. Thymectomy of neonatal animals inhibits the chronic inflammatory response in experimental tumors. A similar effect is observed with the administration of antilymphocytic serum (cytotoxic to thymus-derived T lymphocythes).

The chronic inflammation is greater in tumors composed of virus-transformed cells with persistent presence of virus, than in tumors with no identifiable viral markers.

It is important to note that thymosin is a thymus extracted substance that influences bone-marrow-derived cells (B cells) as postthymic cells. Bone marrow uncommitted cells develop cell surface antigen, characteristic of thymus-derived cells after being treated with thymosin. Bach et al. suggested in 1975 that thymosin may act as a derepressor on the B cells, and by activating B cells to function as mature T cells.

Life Span of Lymphocytes

The life span of lymphocytes varies from days to years. Radiation changes have been observed in peripheral blood lymphocytes ten years after ending radiation therapy. The possibility of permanent irreversible chromosomal changes exists, affecting the lymphocytes to be carried over from one lymphocytic generation to another. Therefore, lymphocytes, with persistent radiation changes, may not necessarily have to be the original ones.

Immunecompetence of the Fetus

When intact, cell-mediated immunity (CMI) can reject a skin graft; but when deficient, there is no rejection. The well-known graft-versus-host (GVH) develops in CMI-competent patient transplanted with poor or leukocyte-free graft of the skin, kidney, or heart. The host's circulating leukocytes, attracted by the foreign tissue, attack the transplant, causing tissue rejection and destruction within two weeks.

The pathogenicity of incompatible transplants is indisputable. Who can deny that small chain of foreign proteins gradually and persistently incorporated into the blood stream is not going to produce a chronic subclinical immune response that years later will manifest in the form of a chronic degenerative disease? For example, fragments of undigested proteins are absorbed into the circulation due to alterations of the stomach lining.

Macrophages are the prominent cells in cell-mediated immunity (CMI). Why the macrophages, and not any other cell, the plasma cell for example? The plasma cell is a function-defined cell, while the macrophage and its precursors, as primitive cells, have totipotential ability. These primitive cells can engulf not only debris and wastes, but also they can differentiate and participate in tissue repair and regeneration.

Since cell-mediated immunity is related to small lymphocytes and these are found in the peripheral blood, examination of the blood by various means gives an indication of the degree of the patient's immunity—for example, the determination of the ratio between the T-helper (T_h) and the T-suppressor (T_m) cells. The greater the number of the T-helper cells, the better the immune system will respond. Lymph nodes biopsies are another way to evaluate the immune system, among other tests.

Chapter III

Cancer and Oncogenic Viruses

The DNA of bacteria and viruses can interact in innumerable ways and change the inheritable characteristic of the organism affected. The liberated viral DNA or viral RNA forms the viral carcinogens. German has stated, "The difference between a virus-induced or a chemical-induced tumor is reported to be due to a distortion of the host DNA by the chemical, while in the virus-induced tumor there is the possible incorporation of a functional segment of viral DNA."

Davis and Parkenson felt that the specificity of the bacterial and viral DNA integration depends on the virus-coded enzyme. "That this enzyme may cut both chains of the DNA of both chromosomes and rejoin them: bacterial to viral and viral to bacterial.

Investigation of electron photographs of DNA molecules achieved by annealing complementary nucleotide chains of various deletion mutants and normal lambda, they concluded that the host (bacterial) and viral integrating sites were not likely to have a nucleotide sequence of more than twelve.

Campbell postulated that during the integration process, there must be an opening of the lambda DNA and that there is a specific insertion point in the host chromosome, thus forming a lineal molecule.

Since DNA hybridization is used to map genes, could this phenomenon happen spontaneously in vivo, thus resulting in evolution or de-evolution?

Most cancers appear as the result of a virus-induced DNA change. Transformed cells in tissue culture show characteristics of cancer cells, but they will not necessarily produce cancer if transplanted into animals or humans. Why is this so? Is it necessary for the host to be cancer prone (genetic predisposition), and is it also necessary to have the proper environment and promoters in order for the cancer to develop?

Human c-Myc gene was identified by using antisera to human myc oncogene. Alterations of the c-Myc gene found in the cell nucleus are related to cell malignant transformation. A similar oncogene, v-Myc, was found in avian myelomatosis (avian leukemia).

Yeasts, fruit flies, rodents, and humans—has an oncogene, ras gene, capable of producing and transforming protein. This protein acts as an activator for the enzyme adenylate cyclase in yeast. Adenylate cyclase plays a fundamental part in the membrane receptors and in cell communication, perhaps even in enhancing the cancer-effector potential of the environment.

The ras genes were first identified in animal cancer viruses that had acquired the gene during the course of infection. The genes of cancer viruses can cause malignant transformation of cells, in contrast with normal genes that do not.

The work of Hsiao, Gattoni-Celli, and Weinstein suggests that the initiating carcinogen may act via activation of a "proto-oncogene." Tumor promoters might stimulate the replication of the transformed cells or complemented the altered cells by activation of other genes. How and where the above takes place is a matter of speculation. It is a known fact that disulfide bonds give stability to the molecular conformation. Do the promoters stimulate the disulfide bonds, thus stabilizing the replication rate of the transformed or cancerous cells?

Abelson murine leukemia virus (Ab-MLV), with the assistance of a C-helper virus, can transform embryo fibroblasts in cell culture, while in vivo it induces a rapid B cell lymphoid leukemia.

Are transplanted tumors rejected by a non-cancer-prone recipient because it is indispensable that the host be cancer prone? If for the occurrence of a virus-induced cancer is necessary that the viral genome integrates with the circular mitochondrial DNA and that both have to be compatible with each other for the integration to occur, then the rejection of the transformed cultures and transplanted cells could be explained, if the compatibility is not present.

Gene amplification is an evolutionary process where one or more genes within a chromosome are duplicated. The duplication process can occur few hundred times within cells, producing gene clusters. Thereafter, the amplified genes are capable of translocation to other chromosomes. Also, it should be noted that cultured mammalian cells have a high incidence of gene amplification.

Are the changes occurring in the in-vitro-transformed cells the same as those in the cancer in vivo?

In reviewing the work on Polyoma and SV40, Dulbecco suggested that the occurrence of the integration, under some restriction, may be due to the same enzyme responsible for the DNA replication. If this view is correct, then the ability of the virus to promote its host DNA synthesis results in integration.

Human T cell leukemia associated with HTLV (human T leukemia virus) or closely related viruses (typical C retrovirus) was identified by Gallo and coworkers in 1981. There is a similarity between HTLV and adult T cell types of leukemia and lymphoma. This association strongly favors the cancer-virus connection.

Human cells can carry genes with cancer potential or oncogenes. These oncogenes can normally function until the cell is provoked into malignant transformation.

Several methods of oncogenes activation have been described, such as "point mutation" by alteration of a gene's part by chemicals or radiation, by infection with a retrovirus carrying an oncogene, or by "amplification" with numerous oncogenes replication within a cell. Grace, Klein, and others have demonstrated another way to activate an oncogene by rearrangement of the B cells chromosome resulting in juxtaposition of oncogenes, thus obtaining gene enhancement. They have found such an occurrence in Burkitt's lymphoma. This very significant finding supports the concept of in vivo cell transformation as a way of cancer metastases of spread.

The cancer patient's macrophages, while engulfing the cancer by-products (wastes and cancer cells), could become infected with the cancer cells' oncogenes and thus are transformed in situ into cancer cells. Since plasmids are transferred from bacteria to bacteria, what prevents a similar phenomenon from occurring in humans? Why not the transfer of cancer genetic material, oncogenes, from cancer cells to macrophages during the process of phagocytosis, thus leading to macrophage transformation?

A plasmid is composed of a double helix. Each DNA strand is composed of four nucleotides. Each strand complements each other.

Taylor was the first to demonstrate that the chromosomes of the eukaryotes replicate in numerous segments or replicons. Others have demonstrated chromosomes translocations in human cancers.

Robert Weinberg has stated, "A single oncogene when transferred into normal cell is unable to transform that cell." But Weinberg and colleagues were able to transform cells by combining several genes, such as RES with adenovirus gene or with Myc. While the particular oncogene may be activated in cancer cells, this is not the case in normal cells of the same patient as found in a tumor isolate from a patient with serious cystoadenocarcinoma of the ovary. This cancer contained an activated K-ras gene while the DNA from the patient's normal cells did not have transforming activity.

Oncogenes, cancer causing genes, are variants of genes responsible for regulating the normal cell division and differentiation. Such gene is represented by the sis gene, (Simian sarcoma virus) that has one of the two proteins found in the platelet-derived growth factor (PDGF).

Subsequent to this, another viral oncogene, the ErbB, related to the epidermal growth factor (EGF) has been described. All viral oncogenes originate from cellular genes that the virus integrates during infection.

Once integration occurs, the oncogene can stimulate cell division by coding for a growth factor as the sis gene does, or by coding for an "aberrant growth factor receptor, thus losing its normal control sequences, as the B apparently does."

Human Cell Transformation

Borek and Hall by treating with 400 rads of x-rays, transformed human diploid skin fibroblasts. These transformed cells are capable of growing in agar, and these are also able to form tumors in nude mice. In these experiments, they used B-stradiol to potentiate the transformation of the irradiated fibroblasts.

The x-ray-treated and transformed mammalian cell showed obvious membrane changes by electron microscopy. Other changes also noted were alterations in the Na+ transport system, increased levels of cellular proteases, and incomplete synthesis of gangliosides.

While normal cells eventually died, transformed cells are immortal. These results, reported by Borek et al., were obtained with the hamster embryo line system, by removing the diploid cells from in vivo growth only after few divisions, and after treatment, the transformation and survival rate ere noted in the culture plates.

Borek et al. obtained reduction of the oncogenic effect by using retinoid SOD, a free radical scavenger. No tumor growth was observed if the cultures were kept under hypothyroid conditions.

Oncogenes and Bittner's Particles

Payne and Chubb were the first to note that the RNA viruses' specificity depends on the genetic information of the mammalian and other vertebrate species. This is the basis of the oncogene and the virogenes theory popularized by Huebner and Tadaro. The principle of this theory is that if all the animal genomes contain oncogenes, then the transformation to malignancy of any particular cell depends on whether there is switching of its oncogenes. Therefore, if the virogenes are expressed, there will not only be production, but liberation of the RNA tumor virus from the cell.

Bittner's viral particles are present in the mammary carcinoma of the mouse and are transmitted through the milk to its descendents.

Margurite Vogt and Renato Dulbecco were the first to transform cells into tumor cells by adding polyomavirus to hamsters' embryo fibroblasts (connective tissue cells) cultures in petri dishes. The transformation is due to the virus DNA.

It has been noted that spontaneous tumors have alteration in the Myc gene. Changes in the Myc gene produce a dominant gene expression in the tumor cells. This is due to chromosome translocation that enhances the oncogenicity of the Myc gene. It appears that some oncogenes may work in tandem, whereby manifestation of a particular oncogene depends on the activation of one or more oncogenes.

Reverse Transcriptase

Replication or copy of the DNA is possible by an enzyme, the reverse transcriptase, first theorized by Temin. The oncogenic hypothesis could explain how the carcinogenic substance could promote the transformation of cells that are already cancer prone. Malignant cells with active oncogenes but without a demonstrable virus may have inactive virogenes. What about the possibility of a prion infesting the DNA, mitochondrial or nuclear, and thus initiating the seed for cancer? Will the presence of viral particles be dispensable then? It may be that during the intimate integration, the automatic cell replication sets in with the simultaneous inhibition of the reproduction of the virus or prions. Could the prions be an integral part of our genes as the oncogenes are?

As our lives evolve in a progressively polluted environment, can our contaminated inner environment modify our genes in order to adapt? As our body ages, so perhaps our genes age; and progressively and gradually, our genes degenerate by mutations in an attempt to adapt.

Pollution is all around us—not only in the air, water, and soil, but in the very food we eat, laced with preservatives, chemicals, toxic coloring, and insecticides.

Medawar in his book *The Life Science* mentions that the viruses are recognized because of the cellular pathological changes; however, he continues, "It is quite possible that our cells harbor a number of silent viruses that have already yielded up their store of genetic information, which has been incorporated into the genome of the cell."

If the above is true, then if the virus's genetic information affects our genes, are we in fact able to transmit to our offspring a particular virus-induced disease predisposition? Is it possible that the disease-producing virus may manifest clinical differences depending whether the virus joins with the nuclear or mitochondrial DNA?

The fusion of the viral circular DNA with the mitochondria circular DNA may eliminate the persistence of the virus as such. This can be compared to the fusion between the sperm and the ovum. But while the sperm-ovum fusion results in a total individual, this is not the case in the virus-mitochondrion integration. In the latter, there is an unevenness of the genetic material between the virus and the mitochondrion DNA, and meiosis (elimination of excess genetic material) cannot occur. Therefore, an abnormal unevenness of DNA is retained.

This unevenness may lead to a replication disequilibrium and metabolic chaos resulting in cell transformation and eventually in endless cancer cell replication. Thus, in part, cancer cells replicate constantly, trying to get rid of the excess unpaired DNA and its cellular wastes.

The more uneven the pairing of the DNAs, perhaps the more rapid the cancer cells replicate in an attempt to reach an internal cellular balance without success.

The integration of virus-mitochondria DNAs will provoke the cell to continuously divide in an effort to transform its cellular division from an irregular to a regular diploid, as it occurs in meiosis of the germ cells. But this cannot be accomplished due to the unevenness of the mixed genetic material present in the abnormal fusion between the virus-mitochondria DNAs.

Diseases occur when there is unevenness or other chromosomal anomalies. Diploid cells go through meiosis in order to reduce the number of chromosome in preparation to fuse with the opposite sex cell. But in virus integration, this phenomenon of meiosis does not happen. Therefore, an abnormal process is initiated resulting in cell transformation and endless division.

Plasma Cells, Antigens, and Antibodies

It has been demonstrated that plasma cells produce specific antigens. If highly radioactive, antigen is injected into an animal, and days later, thin sections of antibody-producing tissue are studied by auroradiographic procedure. Most of the labeled antibodies are found in the macrophages. The plasma cells do not contain any antigen, but few antigens are found in the plasma blasts.

The fact that most of the antibodies are found in the macrophages is very significant. Are the macrophages, which are totipotential cells, then being primed by the antibodies? Does this result into a macrophage-plasma-cell transformation with antibody-specific forming capabilities?

Antibodies are the mirror images of its antigen at the linkage point for the sake of compatibility. B cells stimulated by an antigen react to it by manufacturing a mirror image or a reverse form of the antigen, an antibody. It creates a "lock and key match."

With the production of the antibody, there is an alteration of the cellular steady state. Similar alteration is observed during the virus-chromosome fusion. The feedback mechanism is altered, thus the infected cell cannot "turn off" the viral stimulation to replicate. Once effective, the viral infection is initiated. There is alteration of the remarkable stability of the DNA and of its information. Therefore, transcription is altered. Since each molecule is different, there is a need for complementary fusion zone, where the complementary amino acids facilitate the linkage. If not, then the virus cannot integrate, or it will remain dormant, or the antigen does not bind the antibody due to the lack of specificity.

Alteration of amino acids sequence of a molecule can produce marked biological changes as the alterations observed in hemoglobin resulting in sickle cell disease. In sickle cell disease, two molecules of the amino acid valine replace two molecules of glutamic acid normally present in the normal hemoglobin. This change in a molecule of about six hundred amino acids results in the sickle cell trait or disease depending on the heterozygocyty or homozygocyty inherited.

This amino acid alteration inhibits the hemoglobin from proper arrangement with other hemoglobin molecules, and it results in the formation of precipitation of the hemoglobin molecules in the form of crystals within the red cells when there is reduction in the blood oxygenation. The precipitated hemoglobin crystals deform the RBCs in the form of a sickle and thus the name sickle cell. The alteration results not only in morphologic and physiologic changes in the molecule, but in the RBCs as well.

If the change of two amino acids can produce such a devastating morphologic and physiologic changes, then, how much more drastic changes can produce the fusion of the virus/cell DNAs.

Monoclonal Antibodies

Antibody-secreting cells (plasma cells) can be made immortal by fusing them with tumor cells, and then cloning the hybrids. Highly specific antibodies are then produced by each clone. In 1975, Milstein and colleagues fused mouse myeloma cells with lymphocytes from the spleen of a specifically immunized mouse. The result was a hybrid myeloma or "hybridoma." These cells expressed the immortality of the myeloma cells, and the specificity of antibody production of the lymphocytes.

Hybridization of DNA Molecules

Hybridization of DNA molecules is based on the pairing and rewinding ability of the two DNA strands at the complementary regions to form double helices.

The same amount of DNA is found in all somatic or diploid cells of the same organism. This is not modified by diet or environment. However, when one considers the cellular changes occurring in viral infections and particularly in virus-induced cancer cells, a question that comes to mind is does viral infections alter the individual genetic makeup?

Biosynthesis of the Nucleotides

Buchanan and colleagues fed birds with various isotope-labeled purine possible precursors. When the birds excreta was analyzed, it revealed that the atoms of the purine ring originated as follows: carbon two and eight were provided by the formate, carbon six by CO_2, three nitrogen atoms, and nine arose from the amide group of glutamine, nitrogen one from aspartate, and nitrogen seven from glycine. By these experiments, they were able to find out how the building up of the purine ring occurs step by step, resulting in the formation of the nucleotides. For a detailed explanation see Lehninger's Biochemistry.

The coenzyme tetrahydrofolic acid is the reduced form of folic acid. Tetrahydrofolate (FH4) acts as an intermediate carrier of formyl (-CHO), methyl (-CH3) or hydroxymethyl (-CH2OH) groups in numerous enzymatic reactions. FH4 acts as an intermediate carrier of one carbon transfer related to the metabolism of the purines, pyrimidines, and amino acids. Reduction in folic acid results in inadequate biosynthesis of the pyrimidines, thymines, and purines.

There are enzymes capable or repairing the DNA molecules as long as the complementary strands are intact. This function is important since damage to the DNA in vivo can occur in a single or double strand by shear forces of bending. Local pH changes can produce losses of the purine bases, and x-rays or radiation may affect a base. Similar changes can be obtained with chemicals.

The cells have protective mechanism of DNA repair. One such repair mechanism is the recombination, whereby the damaged segment of DNA is duplicated and replaced by part of the corresponding intact segment of another DNA molecule.

The bacteria E. coli, for example, has an enzyme called ligase. This enzyme can join the ends of the DNA chains. It is present not only in bacteria, but also in eukaryotic cells. The cells utilize this mechanism to repair some DNA damages.

The enzymatic photoreaction mechanism is stimulated by visible blue light illumination of the cell. This process depends upon the enzyme that joins to the defective DNA site. The light activates the enzyme. This mechanism can be used to repair the DNA damaged by ultraviolet light.

There is another mechanism of repair independent of light—"dark" repair, and called excision repair. This repair is dependent upon sequential action of four enzymes. It utilizes polymerases and ligases. Because of its action, it has been called "cut, patch, cut, and seal 'repair'."

Mitochondrial Filaments

Mitochondrial filaments are not a normal occurrence. It has been observed in large abnormal hepatocytes and in various abnormal tissues. The photosynthetic apparatus of the blue-green algae, gleocapsa, are represented by elongated parallel photosynthetic membranes. Does the mitochondrial filament observed in abnormal liver tissue represent the elongated parallel photosynthetic membranes observed in the blue-green algae? Does the energy store house mitochondria in diseases of the animal kingdom, transform its metabolism into a primitive energy-generating system such as observed in the protozoan blue-green algae?

CHAPTER IV

Photosynthesis, Chlorophyll, Chloroplasts, Bacteria Associated with Cancer

The blue-green algae strongly absorb the red light near the water surface. In contrast, the more penetrating blue and green light are absorbed by algae found in deep waters, such as the red and brown algae.

Brown algae use Chlorophyll c and fucoxanthin to absorb light, while blue and green algae utilize Chlorophyll a in more superficial waters.

Photosynthesis

Emerson and Arnold in 1931 and 1932 suggested that the photosynthetic function of chlorophyll is a joint action of many chlorophyll molecules converting a photon into an electron.

A photosynthetic unit is composed of the photoreaction unit—chlorophyll, the antennae, auxiliary pigments, and electron transport chains.

There are various forms of chlorophyll, each adapted for a particular function. For example, while Chlorophyll a is a dimer (two molecules), Chlorophyll b is a trimer in the same circumstances. Chlorophyll b has two donor groups: a formyl group and a keto group.

Green plants, by photosynthesis, transform radiant energy into chemical compounds for their growth. The product of photosynthesis supplies a great percentage of the chemical energy used by other organisms. The exception is some bacteria that obtain their energy from iron or sulfur, thus releasing the chemical energy present in metals and in minerals.

Plants trap the sun's energy and transform it into not only chemicals and nutrients, but also, as a waste product, oxygen, which is essential for life. I propose that plants produce, as a waste product, an active form of oxygen, ozone (O_3), in such a reactive form that quickly changes to oxygen (O_2) upon elimination by the plant. Thus, our atmosphere is replenished of oxygen.

Two kinds of chlorophyll are found in higher oxygen-producing plants: Chlorophyll a and Chlorophyll b. But nonoxygen producing plants do not have Chlorophyll a. The effective absorption of the visible light depends on the chlorophyll-conjugated double bonds. The absorption maxima of an acetone extract of pure Chlorophyll a is at 663 and 420 nm.

One of the discoverers of oxygen, Joseph Priesly, did some of the original experiments on the exchange of matter during photosynthesis in the years 1770–1777. He proved the depletion of oxygen by a burning candle in sealed container. The oxygen in the container could be restored by a sprig of mint over a period of time, and it could support the oxygen needs of a mouse. Therefore, Priestly concluded that green plants evolve oxygen, the reverse process of animal respiration where oxygen is consumed.

Most of the photosynthetic bacteria are strict anaerobic, and use hydrogen sulfide as the electron donor instead of water. All other photosynthetic organisms use water from which molecular oxygen develops. Instead of chloroplasts, photosynthetic bacteria and blue-green algae have membrane-derived structures as their light receptor system.

Photosynthesis in Plants and in Bacteria

Photosynthesis in plants: $H_2O + CO_2$—light = $(CH_2O) + O_2 (O_3)$*

Photosynthesis in bacteria and algae: $2H_2O + CO_2$—light = $(CH_2O) + 26$

* Arnan's modification

Photosynthesis is the transformation of the light energy into chemical energy by the chlorophyll in the chloroplasts. The chemical energy is ATP and other reducing agents. The end result of photosynthesis is the production of carbohydrates and oxygen, but I propose that instead of oxygen (O2), the superoxide ozone (O_3), is produced and it is quickly released as a waste product into the atmosphere where it is transformed into oxygen.

Chloroplasts

In 1880, G. Engelman discovered that the eukaryotic algae spirogyra attracted oxygen-dependent motile bacteria toward its "single large spiral chloroplast," but only when the cell was illuminated. He concluded that the chloroplast was the site of oxygen production because of the attraction of the aerophilic bacteria to the chloroplast site.

Chloroplasts, mitochondria, and viruses have circular DNA in the form of dimers. Chloroplasts and mitochondria are self-replicating, but the virus depends on the host cell for its replication.

Chloroplasts are larger than mitochondria, and therefore, they are easier to isolate. Chloroplasts contain flattened membrane sacs and parallel membranes called thylakoids, and intergranal lamellae respectively. These elements are comparable to the cristae of the mitochondria. It is at the thylakoids and intergranal lamellae where photosynthesis is performed.

Phases of Photosynthesis

Photosynthesis has two phases—a light dependent or light phase, and a dark phase, not light dependent. The photosynthetic reactions occur in the chloroplast. The chloroplasts, as the mitochondria, are complete respiratory units. The light reactions occur during the day or when plants are exposed to the light. The dark reactions can occur both at night and during daytime.

An important characteristic of the light reactions of photosynthesis is the net flow of electrons in the direction of the system having the lower or more electronegative standard potential. "It is the energy of the absorbed light that causes the electrons to flow in reverse, in the direction of the more energy-rich state, opposite to the direction of the electrons flow in respiration."

Similarly in cancer, there must be a reverse electron flow since the cells have changed their metabolism from respiration to fermentation. Therefore, cancer cells appear to have a plantlike physiology.

Transformation of cell from normal cell to a cancer cell cannot occur unless this change has taken place. It is necessary for the cell to be transformed in order to change from a respiratory animal-cell physiology to a plant-cell physiology. Cancer cells cannot produce superoxide dismutase or ozone (O_3) as normal cell do. Therefore, cancer cells cannot get rid of their wastes readily.

The principal chlorophyll of higher plants is Chl a. It has a green color because it absorbs red and blue lights and transmits green light. The maximum absorption of red light is at 665 nm and for the blue light is 430 nm. Chlorophyll b's maximum red absorption is 645 nm instead of 665 nm.

With the absorption of a quanta of light, the chlorophyll molecule, becomes excited, loses an electron, and becomes positive charged.

Chlorophyll and cytochromes are porphyrins, but chlorophyll has a magnesium molecule, Mg++, in the center of the porphyrin instead of an iron, Fe++, as found in the hemoglobin molecule.

Cancer and Superoxide Dismutase

The absence of superoxide dismutase in SV40-transformed embryonic cells was reported by N. Yamanaka and D. Deamer in 1974. Dionisi et al. found absence or minimal amount of superoxide dismutase activity in the hepatoma mitochondria. They concluded that lack of superoxide dismutase in tumors may be a general characteristic.

There is instant and rapid synthesis of mitochondria DNA when anaerobic yeasts are exposed to oxygen, however, the synthesis level decrease after ten minutes of exposure to oxygen.

Available evidence supports the view that cancer cells and other anaerobic organisms cannot survive for a long period of time in an oxygenated environment, and therefore, they lack the structures and the ability to produce oxidative enzymes and cannot oxidize.

Chlorophyll

Chlorophyll, the metal-porphyrin molecule, found in green plants and blue-green algae, has magnesium (Mg^{++}) at the center of the porphyrin ring, instead of iron (Fe^{++}), as found in the hemoglobin molecule. Iron cannot carry on photosynthesis, as pointed out by Calvin.

Heme portion of hemoglobin molecule. Notice central Iron (Fe^{++}).

Chlorophyll c molecule. Notice the central magnesium (Mg ++).

Porphyrin is a pigment compound widely distributed in nature. It consists of four pyrrol nuclei joined into a ring structure. This nucleus has the ability to combine with various metals such as iron, magnesium, copper, and others, and with nitrogenous substances. It is to be noted that porhyrin pigment fluoresces as chlorophyll does.

Chlorophyll, by capturing a quantum of solar energy, mediates energy migration and utilization with great efficiency, through the prolonged excitation of magnesium. This cannot be done with iron because of its natural magnetism. However, in the animal kingdom, iron is indispensable for numerous enzymatic activities including the breaking down of hydrogen peroxide (H_2O_2) to water and oxygen, (H_2O and O_2).

Iron is necessary for the combination of the enzyme catalase with hydrogen peroxide. In the hemoglobin molecule, the porphyrin ring contains in its center iron instead of magnesium. Iron is responsible for the transportation of oxygen by the hemoglobin in the red blood cells (RBCs).

Chlorophyll Fluoresces

The fluorescent activity of the chlorophyll can be enhanced in a saline solution at high glycerol concentration, as reported by L. A. Staehelin and A. J. Arntzen in the Ciba Foundation Symposium # 61, 1979, p.166.

I have found in my laboratory experiments that when living cancer cells are suspended in normal saline solution, and are observed by the light microscopy, there was the production of green granules (GG) within the cancer cell's cytoplasm. The GG appeared in the cancer cells after being exposed to the light for few minutes. Similar control suspension of cancer cells kept in the dark for an equal amount of time did not show green granules (GG). But the GG appeared after few minutes of light exposure. What photochemical reaction stimulates the appearance of the GG? Are the primitive cancer cells reverting to a plantlike physiology when exposed to the light?

As has been mentioned before, there is a similarity between the hemoglobin (blood pigment) and the chlorophyll (plant pigment), and interestingly enough, they are complimentary colors—one red and the other green.

During the live cycle, plants utilize the animal kingdom's waste products, such as urea in the form of nitrogen and carbon dioxide (CO_2), to live and to produce food that the animal kingdom utilizes for survival. At the same time, plants eliminate oxygen (O_2 or O_3*), indispensable for animal life, and the animal kingdom, in return eliminates carbon dioxide (CO_2) that plants use for photosynthesis. Is nature telling us something? Perhaps, to have a long and healthy life, we should eat complementary food from the plant kingdom, instead of food from the animal kingdom?

Should we try to avoid food products of animal origin? Because of their chemical resemblance to our body's composition, they could start a gradual and persistent autoimmune process, such as aging, predisposition to infectious diseases, arthritis, skin diseases, artherosclerosis, multiple sclerosis, and other degenerative diseases including cancer and acquired immune deficiency syndrome (AIDS). Was the forbidden fruit in the Garden of Eden a particular kind of protein?

With inadequate digestion due to an inadequate amount of digestive enzymes and with a concomitant inflammatory process in the bowel or stomach, exogenous protein material in the form of a chain of amino acids can be absorbed into the circulation and initiate an immune response to the foreign protein, thus planting the seed to an endless and chronic degenerative process. According to the individual predisposition, this process may later on manifest as multiple sclerosis, scleroderma, arthritis, and others.

If the animal product is in close composition to the individual or other animal eating it, is the antibody stimulation greater?

Photosynthesis is not only important for food production, but for the natural production of oxygen essential for our survival. Therefore, to obtain ecological balance, it is indispensable to care for and protect our forests. Indiscriminate cutting of trees and contamination of our environment with insecticides and other dangerous chemicals result in a drastic alteration of our environment's steady state, thus resulting in a negative balance. The end result of this chaos jeopardizes life on Earth.

Photosynthesis is dependent on light and temperature. The rate of photosynthesis is proportional to the intensity of light and temperature. But while the chemical reactions in photosynthesis are temperature dependent, the light reactions are not.

It was F. F. Blackman, an English biologist, who in 1905 discovered and labeled the light and the dark reactions of photosynthesis.

Photosynthesis is a synthesizing process requiring energy. With the help of a reducing agent, nicotinamide adenine dinucleotide phosphate (NADPH), carbon dioxide (CO_2) is converted into complex organic molecules. The energy supplied by ATP is formed from the diphosphate ADP plus phosphate.

When a molecule of chlorophyll is hit by light, an electron is kicked out of the orbital of the chlorophyll molecule. A reduction and an oxidation capability develop. It is the strong oxidizing capability of the chlorophyll (Chl+) that generates the molecular oxygen by oxidation of water. Therefore, during the photochemical reactions, NADPH, ADP, ATP, and molecular oxygen are produced.

These previously described steps of photosynthesis are light dependent, but the formation of carbohydrates by reduction of CO_2 is not light dependent and can occur in the dark.

Kenyon and Steinman demonstrated the formation with polymerization of macromolecules to photocells in an ascending graph, starting from simple compounds of H, C, O, and N, and followed by intermediate organic matter (amino acids, etc.).

Subsequently, they found that there was a formation of polymers with the progressive formation of cell membrane. The polymers had an anaerobic metabolism. This was represented graphically. The upper part of the graph illustrated the more advanced forms of fermentation. Later on, they discovered the appearance of pigmented cells with photosynthetic ability, respiration, and release of CO_2.

Miller, Urey, and Oparin made observations on the formation of amino acids from basic elements. In the observation of Miller, amino acids were formed by mixing ammonia, hydrogen, cyanide, and aldehyde when exposed to an electrical current is fundamental.

All of this give us hints as to how organized matter can be formed from simple molecules by plants and animals, and how under the influence of electrical current, simple molecules can get arranged into amino acids and other compounds.

The Role of Light in Nature

Light can be described as an electromagnetic radiation in the form of packages or quanta (a quantum is a unit of radiant energy), as first suggested by a German physicist Max Planck in 1900. A few years later, in 1905, Albert Einstein provided an explanation resting on the theory that the electromagnetic radiation comes in packages or quanta. The energy, in one quantum of electromagnetic radiation, is proportional to its frequency.

At the turn of the century, it was observed that there was a photoelectric effect when shining a light on a metal surface. This resulted in the ejection of electrons from the metal surface. It was also noted that there was a lower limit in which the light can effectively produce the emission of the photoelectrons.

Cordes and Schaeffer wrote that "one quantum of light may strike one atom and, if it has sufficient energy, and hence a low energy per quantum (red light), and if this energy is less than the energy required to kick out one electron, the photoelectric effect cannot occur regardless of the number of the quanta that strike the metal." Therefore, there is a threshold of energy for the photoelectric effect.

Albert Einstein, in 1905, acknowledged the basic relationship of energy and matter. He defined this in the formula $E=mc^2$. His formulation revolutionized physics and is considered fundamental in science.

If an electron, (an electronegative particle of ether revolving around the positive proton forming an atom), and a positron (an anti-electron, positive electron) collide, the electron and the positron disappear by the process called annihilation. But two gamma rays are formed. Thus, matter has been then transformed into energy. Consequently, matter and energy are two forms of a basic element.

According to the photochemical laws, chemical reactions can occur by the absorption of light by a molecule. The reactions happen only when the light quanta absorbed is effective enough to produce chemical changes.

Fluorescence results from the excitation produced by a photon on a single molecule. Fluorescence is a characteristic of chlorophyll, the plant pigment needed for photosynthesis.

Chlorophyll molecules are organized in arrays for the efficient energy transfer between molecules. The array absorbs the light quanta. The quanta of light may be transported to the reaction site, where the quantum's energy will be utilized to produce chemical changes.

The chemical reactions in photosynthesis are dependent on temperature, while the light reactions are not temperature dependent.

Porphyrins, by absorbing the light energy, pass it to an oxygen molecule producing a very active single oxygen. Since single oxygen reactivity destroys tissue, this is the base of a cancer therapy—phototherapy. Chlorophyll is a porphyrin with central magnesium. Porphyrins are given to cancer patients, and days after, the photosensitized cancer patients are treated with light or phototherapy. The porphyrin-targeted cancerous tissue is selectively destroyed. Hemoglobin, another porphyrin, has iron at its center instead of magnesium, which is present in chlorophyll.

CHAPTER V

Oxygen, Hemoglobin Transport, Bacteria in Cancer Tissues, Macrophages, and Alphafetoprotein

Hemoglobin and Oxygen Transport. Each hemoglobin molecule has an iron carrying element, the heme. It is within the heme attached to the iron molecule where the molecule of oxygen is transported. Since each RBC can carry about 300 million hemoglobin molecules and one hemoglobin molecule can carry eight atoms of oxygen, each RBC can transport 2,400 million atoms of oxygen.

In vertebrates, the RBCs release the CO_2 collected from the tissues and transfer it to the lungs, where, through the delicate alveolar capillary's wall, the CO_2 is expelled going into the atmosphere. In turn, the atmospheric O_2 is retained in the RBCs by the hemoglobin (hb) pigment.

The hemoglobin, while travelling through the capillaries, will in turn release the O_2 to the tissues and collect the CO_2 and other cellular wastes; so the cycle continues.

If the RBCs and other tissue cells are coated by antibodies, the normal exchange of nutrients and elimination of wastes are curtailed or inhibited. Thus, the proper polluted inner environment favorable for any kind of infection or other diseases is created.

The so-polluted body is ready to attract diseases as a flower is ready to be pollinated by offering nectar and attractive colors to insects and birds.

Some of the pathogenic organisms may produce immediate disease while others, depending on the individual remaining resistance, may stay in a dormant stage, awaiting the proper opportunity to thrive. By then, years after the original infestation or sensitization, degenerative diseases may appear according to the individual genetic predisposition.

There is a constant interplay between the genetic component and the environment. If the balance between the two is lost, disease (dis-ease) occurs.

Blood Supply and Cancer

Oxygen is more soluble in cold water. Cancers, in general, are poorly vascularized once they reach a certain size. With radio tracers, the cancerous lesions are called cold nodules due to the absence of the radioactive material in the suspected lesions because of poor vascularization. Cancer creates its proper anaerobic environment by decreasing the number of blood vessels present within and around the tumor. However, cancer needs blood, not to provide oxygen, but nutrients, without which the cancer tissue will die and produce tumor necrosis. This is a frequent finding in large cancers where the central portion of the tumor is too far from the blood vessel to get adequate nutrients and thus necrotizes. However, Gullino has reported on the increased temperature at the tumor site in comparison with the peripheral or contralateral normal tissue. He attributed the increase in temperature to tumor angiogenesis (tumor vascular growth).

Gullino also found the pH of the mammary carcinoma of the mouse to be acidic, pH 6.8. This decreased because the temperature of the tumor was increased. Localized hyperthermia treatment of the tumor produced an increase in the blood flow and oxygenation, but too high a temperature produced vascular collapse.

Another characteristic of cancer is the lack of lymphatic system. Cancer isolates itself from the host-tissue immune system (T lymphocytes).

There is a current trend toward hyperthermia treatment of tumors in the clinical setting. The rationale being that by increasing oxygenation there will be an inhibitory effect on the cancer. However, with increased vascularization of the tumor, there will be a greater amount of nutrients also made available to the tumor. Therefore, this therapeutic modality has to be used in conjunction with other therapies and not by itself.

While it may initially seem to beneficial in some cancers, hyperthermia therapy will do more harm to the patient eventually. The killing of cancer cells in vivo will release cancer proteins and antigenic substances that will stimulate B cells to produce antibodies, and by further activation of the macrophages and subsequent metastases.

In vitro studies of tumor and normal cells exposed to variations in temperature, do not demonstrate significant effect, but cancer cells in vivo appear to be sensitive to heat. This was interpreted to be related to the lower pH, low pO_2, and poor nutrition.

While hyperthermia may initially reduce the tumor size, eventually the tumor growth will recur with renewed speed.

Mycoplasma-like Bodies in Plant and Animal Tissues

Wolanski has described mycoplasma-like bodies in plants and in animal tissues. He has interpreted these bodies as preparation artifacts, since he did not find similar structures in either healthy or diseased plant material that has been pretreated with glutaraldehyde and osmium tetraoxide.

Artifacts similar to those seen in plant extracts can also be produced by PTH staining of the HeLa cells, but not when the material was treated with fixative prior to the negative staining. Are these truly artifacts or inactive bacterial forms ready to multiply and produce disease as soon as there is a decrease in the immunity of the host? At the moment, there is no definite answer.

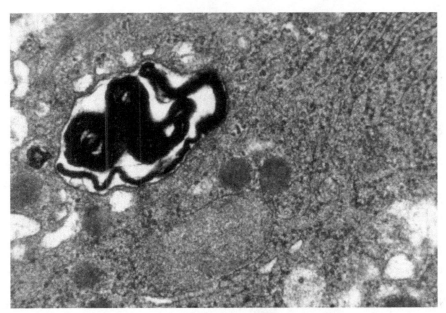

Electron photographed degenerating particle. Human breast cancer.

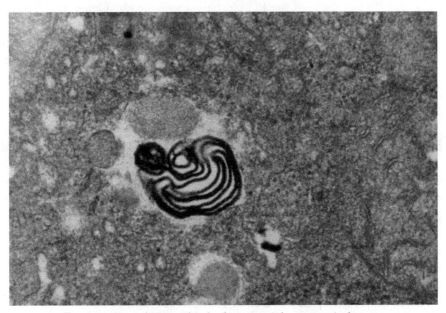

Degenerating pleomorphic body or particle present in human
breast adenocarcinoma (electron photo)

Bacteria Present in Cancer

The question whether microorganisms and viruses are associated and present in cancer tissue is not a new one. Several scientists have reported on its association with cancer. Some such as Metchnikoff, Shope, Rous, and Drs. Virginia Livingston and Eleanor Jackson have reported on microorganisms in cancerous tissue.

Livingston and Jackson isolated a pleomorphic acid-fast microorganism from neoplastic lesions of man and animals. They named this organism Progenitor cryptocides (PC). This organism was also found, not only within the cancer cells, but within the RBCs and WBCs (white blood cells) of cancer patients and of patients with chronic degenerative diseases.

The P. cryptocides was found to fluoresce and to be refractile in certain forms; to be filterable through filters that keep out bacteria; to grow aerobically, microaerophillically or anaerobically; and to have a fetid odor on heavy growth. Vegetative forms of the PC can withstand up to 90°C of heat for fourteen minutes. One of the most striking characteristics of the PC beside its pleomorphism is its ability to produce choriogonadotropin (CGH) in the test tube as described and reported by Dr. Virginia Livingston in 1974. Since then, this characteristic of the PC has been confirmed by Cohen and Stramp and by S. S. Koide.

Livingston emphasizes the significance of the CGH production by the PC, and in her observation, the PC rides on the head of the sperm and its relationship with the fact that the ovum has a CGH receptor. For more detailed information, check the many articles published by Livingston and Jackson on the subject.

When visiting Dr. Livingston at her home and at her laboratory in San Diego, California, she demonstrated to me, by dark field microscopy, the presence of the Progenitor cryptocides within the RBCs and plasma of fresh blood of several cancer patients. While there, I also demonstrated to her saline suspensions of her PC culture under the microscope, and how the colorless pleomorphic bacteria became emerald green in color after few minutes of observation under the light microscope. Is this a photosynthetic phenomenon of the PC?

Subsequently, I have observed in the blood of all my cancer patients, and patients with chronic diseases, as well as apparently healthy persons, the presence of pleomorphic organisms cocci, coccobacilli, rods, and protozoa. There is a direct relationship between the seriousness of the patient's condition and the number of bacteria present. I use this test of live cell analysis to evaluate and follow up all my patients.

If the patient is responding to the treatment, whatever is the condition, the number of bacteria in the blood decreases.

Does the presence of the PC indicate that this microorganism is the cause of cancer or any specific disease condition? There is no conclusive answer yet.

The pleomorphic bacteria, (PC) may be part of our genetic makeup as oncogenes are. These organisms and its genetic predisposition being dormant, as long as the individual is constitutionally strong, have a healthy immune system. Once there is derangement of health status and the steady state is altered by a disease process, all the dormant predispositions may be manifested in the particular individual. If we are made of the "dust of the earth," then we can have within all potential manifestations. The diseased body creates the proper environment for the formation and proliferation of all kind of protozoa, bacteria, or viruses. Their presence becomes obvious and more prominent, according to the particular condition as the disease worsens.

I have studied cancer tissues under light and electron microscope trying to find and identify microorganisms. With special stains such as PAS (periodic acid Schiff) and Gram's, I was able to observe pleomorphic bacteria within cancer cells in cancer of the prostate, and as well as artifacts by electron microscope studies of cancer of the breast and ovary. Notice text illustrations.

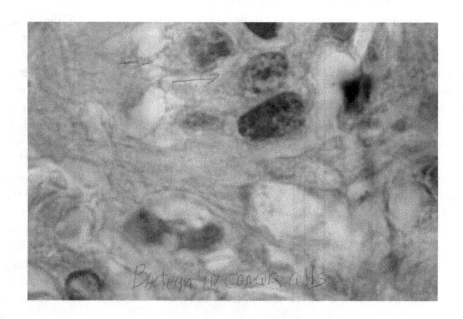

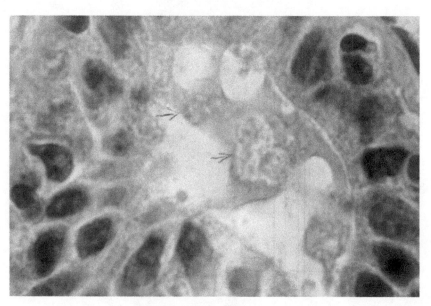

Intracellular bacteria in cancer tissues

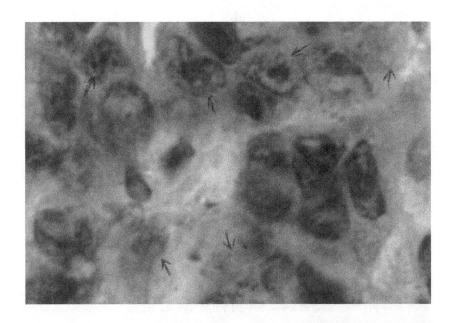

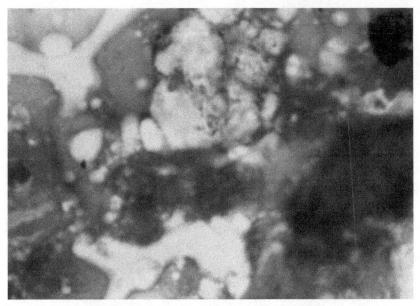

Intracellular bacteria in cancer cells
Intracellular bacteria demonstrated with special stain

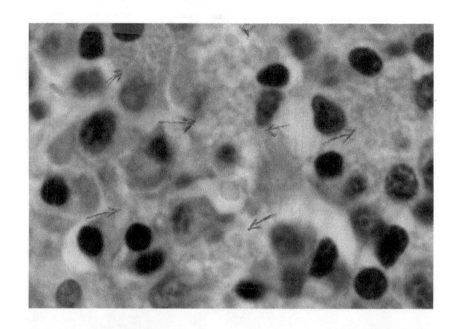

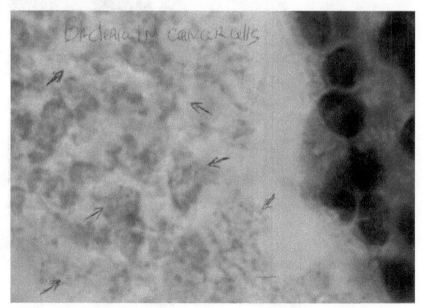

Bacteria present in cancer cells

Chapter VI

Cancer and Nutrition

There is an apparent relationship between a high-protein diet and cancer incidence. For example, in Oriental countries where the usual diet is predominantly vegetarian with sparse animal product supplementation, the incidence of cancer of the colon is lower than that observed in Western countries. This discrepancy gradually disappears when Orientals eat a Westernized diet. The disease predisposing pattern starts manifesting in the second generation of Westernized Orientals.

However, because of the usual association between high levels of fat with a high-protein Western diet, it is difficult to say which of the two, or whether both, protein and fat, are the culprits. Excessive beer drinking has been associated with an increased risk of colorectal cancer.

In 1954, Babson noted acceleration on the growth of transplanted tumors in rats fed with increased dietary casein from none to 18 percent.

White and Andervont observed in 1943 that cystine-deficient casein-diet-fed female C3H mice failed to develop mammary tumors after twenty-two months. However, when cystine was added to the diet, most of the animals developed tumors.

In 1944, White and White noted that lysine-deficient diet decreased the incidence of mammary carcinoma of the C3H mice. The incidence of the tumors were 25 percent while most of the mice developed tumors once the diet was supplemented with lysine. Later, the same researcher described how he enhanced the incidence of three methylcholanthrene-induced leukemia in casein-fed mice supplemented with cystine, but not with lysine and tryptophan.

Kolonel et al. reported in 1981 that in humans there is a significant correlation between the consumption of animal protein and cancer of the prostate, cancer of the breast, and endometrial adenocarcinoma.

Howell in 1974, and Armstrong and Dali in 1975 reported on the relationship of meat intake with prostatic carcinoma and prostatic carcinoma mortality. There is evidence to support the relationship between dietary fat and cancers of the breast, colon, and prostate. In laboratory experiments, there is evidence to the relationship between the high-protein diet and cancer.

It was the opinion of the committee on cancer that cancer is mostly a preventable disease and that there are specific cancer-inducing agents such as tar, nicotine, asbestos, and others associated with certain types of cancers—for example, smoking in association with cancer of the lungs and excessive beer drinking with colonorectal carcinoma.

Experimental limitation of the body weight of mice by caloric restriction resulted in lower incidence of spontaneous mammary tumors, and of induced skin tumors and sarcomas. Tannenbaum suggested that a predisposition to cancer develops in obese people more than in people below or within the normal weight range. Other researchers, by limiting the caloric intake, found inhibition in the development of the spontaneous mammary carcinoma of the C3H mice. Saxton et al. reported that by giving a balanced diet but, in limited amounts, the incidence of leukemia was 10.1 percent in comparison with the controls of the high incidence leukemia of 65 percent in the normally fed controls. They concluded that while the leukemic transformation was delayed, it was not absolutely prevented by underfeeding.

Winich, in the introduction to his book *Nutrition and Cancer*, stated, "Both the quantity and the quality of the dietary fat can influence tumor incidence. Deficiency in lipotropes results in an increased incidence of both, spontaneous and induced liver tumors in rats and in chickens. Although the results are not conclusive, it has been suggested that vitamin A and vitamin C may protect against certain types of tumors." Rather than a carcinogen itself, fat acts as a promoting agent enhancing certain carcinogens.

There is a direct relationship between cigarette smoking and lung cancer. Cancer of the head and neck, esophagus, pancreas, kidney and bladder are also associated with tobacco carcinogens, such as aromatic amines and hydrocarbons.

Food, in general, may contain carcinogens in the form of additives or preservatives, such as nitrites, that can form nitrosamine, a potent carcinogen. Artificial coloring, tar products, and pollution of the water and air all contribute to disease and cancer promotion.

The National Research Council Panel on Cancer recommends changes in diet to reduce the risk of cancer. Some of the recommendations are that the daily food intake should include whole grain cereals, fruits, and vegetables, especially those high in vitamin C and beta-carotene, which is converted by the body into vitamin A. Especial emphasis should be placed on citrus fruits, dark green and yellow vegetables, and on members of the cruciferae such as cabbage, cauliflower, brussels sprouts, and broccoli.

Vitamins and minerals, including selenium, present in these foods inhibits the formation of free radicals and other cancer-promoting chemicals.

The National Research Council Panel (NRCP) also recommends the reduction in consumption of preserved foods, such as smoked, salt cures, and salt pickled because of association with cancers of the stomach and esophagus (e.g., hotdogs, bacon, ham, sausages, smoked fish).

Also recommended is the avoidance of excessive consumption of alcohol. Alcohol, in association with cigarette smoking, increases the risk of cancers of the respiratory and upper gastrointestinal tract, beside other unhealthy conditions, such as bronchitis, hypertension, asthma, emphysema, and laryngitis.

It is suggested to reduce the intake of animal proteins and fat, preferring to eat lean meat and white meat of fowl and fish. Fatty food should be avoided and dietary fiber should be increased to stimulate peristalsis and elimination of wastes.

High-temperature cooking produces mutagens in the food. Caution is to be exercised in food related substances and additives, such as the newly introduced artificial sweetener aspartame. This artificial sweetener is used in many soft drinks, ice cream, sauces, candies, and cakes. There have been reports of dizziness, loss of equilibrium, disorientation, and visual impairment associated with the consumption of aspartame. It appears that during metabolism, aspartame breaks down into methanol or wood alcohol, formaldehyde, and formic acid. Alcohol is not the only responsible for the symptoms, but also damage to the eyes occurs by another by-product of aspartame metabolism, formaldehyde. Formaldehyde is a known carcinogen.

Danger of cancer promotion does not only exist with chemicals, but a new and potentially more dangerous pollution exist with the current research in gene splicing and its possible after effect if human infestation occurs. The very essence of our beings, our genetic code is in danger of contamination and destruction.

Jeremy Rifkin, an environmentalist, fought against experiments in genetic engineering that may endanger our environment. He obtained a restraining order, but it could not be enforced since private companies not regulated by the same laws, were doing similar experiments.

Immunity and Age

There is an apparent reduction in immunity in the two extremes of life ages—in the very young and in the very old.

Statistics of death in children show that there is a forty-fold incidence of neuroblastoma in children up to three months of age. It is a well-known fact of the increased cancer incidence in the old age.

Leukemias and lymphomas incidences is are increased in patients with immunodeficiency and diseases such as Chédiack-Higashi anomaly, ataxia telangectasia, Hodgkin's disease, and the Bruton type agammaglobulinemia to name a few. Jausset, in 1926, reported a decreased frequency of delayed positive hypersensitive skin reactions to tuberculin in adults.

Infections and Cancer

Cancer patients have a progressive inability to fight bacterial, fungal, or viral infections. This may be due, in part, to the leukopenia present in treated patients, or to the suppression of the immune system by the cancer antigen. This antigen leads to an immune paralysis, and to a lack of immune response to any other antigen but the cancer antigen.

Consequently, infections such as pneumonia, urinary tract infections, septicemia, and soft tissue infections are frequent complications in cancer patients.

Most of the bacterial infections are due to gram-negative bacteria, including Psedomona aeruginosa, E. coli, and the Klebsiella-Enterobacter group. These infections are particularly significant in patients under chemotherapy and/or immunosuppressive drugs. Fungal infections are found, not only in leukemic cases, but also in patients with solid tumors under chemotherapy. The most frequent pathogens are from the Aspergillus and Candida species. Pneumocystis carinii pneumonia is found in extremely immunosuppressed patients such as AIDS patients, where this type of pneumonia is a frequent cause of death. Viral infections are frequently associated with cancer in the form of herpes and others.

Dysproteinemias

Multiple myeloma, heavy chain disease and Waldenstr m's macroglobulinemia are dysproteinemias with abnormal findings in the immunoglobulins IgG, IgA and IgM. If immunoglobulins or antibodies protect us against diseases, then what went wrong with the protective mechanism that infections incur in spite of the excessive amount of antibodies present?

Are the antibodies the answer to our general health protection? Or are the antibodies, in general, the direct cause of diseases? Are the antibodies the good guys or the bad guys?

There is supporting evidence that there is a close interplay between cancer pathogenesis and immunology. M. G. Lewis and coworkers demonstrated that patients with malignant melanoma had in their sera antibodies against tumor cells. They also found that there was some antibody specificity, and that in occasion, these antibodies reacted "against the surface membrane of the living autologous tumor cells."

They also found, by immunofluorescence or complement-dependent cytotoxicity, these antibodies are predominantly found in the early and localized stages of the tumor growth. The antibodies become detectable once the widespread of metastases is just to occur.

Lewis and coworker suggested that there is a derangement of the immune regulation system with the production of anti-antibodies or immunocomplexes, rather than immunodeficiency in cancer patients.

I strongly support their view and advice against immunostimulation since the end result will be counterproductive. In my electron microscope studies of concentrate of the globulin fraction of a patient with carcinomatosis, there were innumerable immunocomplexes. It is my impression that the immunocomoplexes, not only coat the normal cells surfaces, thus inhibiting the normal metabolic exchanges, but also clog the circulatory system—venous, arterial, and lymphatic.

As the vicious cycle continues, progressive derangement of the organs occurs—the kidney may be clogged with immunocomplexes, therefore proper filtration is impaired; the blood levels of the liver enzymes may increase because of improper oxygenation, and so on.

Furthermore, I propose that the whole immune system of the cancer patient is so oversaturated and sensitized to the cancer antigen that it is unable to respond to any other immunologic stimulus with adequacy. Therefore, a cancer patient is not immunologically protected and eventually succumbs to various infections in spite of an hyperactive immunoblastic anticancer response, but with no room to respond to any other antigen, but to the cancer antigen alone.

The apparent immunological paralysis is not due to deficiency of the immune system, but to overstimulation and oversaturation of the immune system, thus rendering it unable to respond to any other stimulus, but the cancer antigen.

Svet-Moldavsky et al. reported on tumor growth inhibition, and found that except for the mammary adenocarcinoma that grew in newborn and in adult mice, all other transplanted tumors failed to grow in the newborn mice or there was a retarded growth response, while it grew readily in the adult mice.

Is the lack of a well developed immune system (immunoblasts, plasmacells, etc.) in the newborn mice responsible for the transplanted tumor's growth failure? Does cancer growth depend on the immune competence of the host? Since there is no immune response, there will be no antibody production that I feel is essential for cancer growth. This could explain the failure of transplanted cancer to thrive in newborn mice, and its rapid growth when cancer is transplanted into an adult mouse with a responsive and fully developed immune system, capable of producing immunoglobulin or antibodies—cancer nutrient.

Studying mammary adenocarcinoma of the C3H/HEJ mice and of various human cancers, including cancer of the breast, papillary adenocarcinoma of the ovary, squamous carcinoma of the lung, adenocarcinoma of the colon and melanoma of the skin, I found, by electron microscopy, the presence of immunocomplexes scattered about every area of the tissue. Immunocomplexes were also observed coating the RBC membranes and vacuoles within the cancer cells.

Localized Antigenic Stimulation

In 1922, Davies reported the presence of high titer of specific anti-Shigella agglutinins in the stools of patients with bacillary dysentery within the first twenty-four to thirty-six hours, while at that time no antibodies could be found in the serum.

Ogra reported in 1969, that when children were immunized with live polio vaccine, the antigenic stimulation remained localized to the original stimulated site.

Haremans and Bazin found, by oral immunization with horse spleen ferritin to germfree mice, that "most of the cells containing anti-FRT were located in the mucosa of the intestine (excluding Payer's patches), and their antibody belonged to the IgA class." They also found, after thirty days of immunization, that there was a weak titer of IgA circulating anti-FRT antibodies. While antibody-mediated immunity depends upon five different immunoglobulins—IgG, IgA, IgM, IgD, and IgE, for the body's humoral defense, all are related to the B cells or plasma cells.

The cell-mediated immune response (CMI) depends upon the interaction between the immunogen to stimulate the T cells of the lymphocytic series to produce lymphokinins that may help destroy virus infected cells. This in turn activates the macrophages to participate in the virocidal and phagocytic activity.

It is known that viruses such as the adenovirus, toxins and hormones bind to specific cell membrane receptors, and that the bound attached site gets into the cells through membrane pore or pits and is digested in endosomes. This phenomenon may serve as a sensitizer. Continuation of such an attack may promote cell transformation.

CHAPTER VII

Free Radicals, Oxygen, and Ozone

Dr. Lester Packer, director of the Bioenergetics Group at the University of California at Bekerley, told at a scientific workshop on oxygen radicals in reference to oxygen, "We can't live without it and we can't live indefinitely in its presence." Free radicals are formed constantly during the normal metabolic processes but are destroyed or neutralized by the enzymes system. If the enzymes system is ineffective, there will be damage to the cells. This damage can progressively lead to aging and disease.

The discoverer of the vitamin C and Nobel laureate Dr. Albert Szent-Gyorgi, scientific director of the National Foundation for Cancer Research, explains the role of methoxyhydroquinone (MHQ) in cellular metabolism. "Oxygen is activated by MHQ which in turn oxidizes ascorbic acid to dehydroascorbic acid. These substances form a reversible redox system, the electrochemical potential of which has been measured." It is hypothesized that the absence of this chain distinguishes a cancer cell from a healthy cell.

Ozone

Ozone (O_3) is an activated form of oxygen (O_2). By its oxidizing ability, it neutralizes free radicals and waste products, facilitating their elimination. Ozone is a bluish gas produced in nature during thunderstorms. It is also produced with electric sparks in an oxygenated atmosphere. Thus, it was first noticed in 1883 by Van Marum while experimenting with electrostatic machine. Years later, in 1840, Schonbein submitted a paper to the Munich Academy of Sciences stating that there was a strange-smelling substance produced by the oxygen released during electrolytic dissociation of water.

Ozone (O_3) was used during World War I to treat gangrene and to neutralize bad odors. Currently, O_3 is being used for water purification in the United States and European countries such as Germany, Austria, and Italy. It is utilized in medicine to treat conditions in which improved oxygenation is required.

Ozone is also produced by ultraviolet lamp, radioactive emission, and cathode rays. The oxidation of phosphorus produces O_3. Adenosinetriphosphate (ATP) is manufactured in the mitochondria, and it is indispensable to health. Does ATP produce ozone during normal physiology since it has three molecules of phosphorus? If it does produce O_3, then the detoxification of the cell with neutralization of the cell's wastes can be explained.

German researchers R. Viebahn and others explain the O_3 action on activation of the cellular enzymal protection system against peroxides, activation of the erythrocytic metabolism and an increase of 2,3-DPG, and by a direct influence of the O_3 on the redux function of the mitochondrial respiratory chain, as explained by Viebahn as an example, the significant reduction in NADH. All of these result in improved tissue oxygenation.

Also, the blood flow can be increased due to the action of ozone on freeing the antibody-coated RBCs from its antibodies, thus reducing the tendency of the RBCs to rouleaux formation. With the elimination of antibodies, the normal flexibility of the RBCs and the cellular exchanges are restored.

Since cancer cells are poorly equipped with enzymes, they have no protection against ozone. Thus, ozone produces a metabolic imbalance in malignant cells.

Brinkman et al., in 1958, reported their work with ozone as a possible radiomimetic gas. Muller and coworker found a good tumor response by administering O_3 intravenously to patients with gynecological cancers also receiving radiotherapy. They interpreted that the O_3 had a synergistic effect on the radiation therapy resulting in a better tumor response to the treatment.

In 1973, Teake et al., studied the effect of ozone on the growth of tumors and the effect of irradiation. Cotruvo et al., in 1977, investigated the mutagenic effects of products of ozonations in water. Heinz Konrad, at the Sixth Ozone World Congress in 1983, held in Washington DC, presented his clinical experience treating two small groups of patients—one group with herpes, and the other group with viral hepatitis, type A, type B, and type non-A-non-B. His conclusion was that ozone, "though not being the only possible approach to these diseases, is the best approach, mainly because of its fast results, and because of its safety and the absence of undesirable effects."

At the same ozone congress, Dr. Rokitansky summarized his clinical and biochemistry studies of ozone therapy in peripheral arterial circulatory disorders, with the statement that "the curative effect of intravascular ozone therapy is the significant increase in 2,3-DPG. This facilitates the release of oxygen from hemoglobin."

Dr. Horst Wermeister of Germany reported on the good response obtained by treating two hundred cases of therapy-resistant ulcerations. By using oxygen-ozone gas treatments under negative pressure, the chronic ulcers healed, where other standard therapies had failed. Other successful treatments were reported by Dr. Fritz Kramer, DDs from Germany; he used ozone as a disinfectant. Satisfactory results were reported by Dr. Derlef Hofman and others in the use of oxygen-ozone therapy in coronary disease.

Robert Meyer, MD, a pediatrician from Florida, presented two papers—one on his animal experiments, and the other, on his clinical experience with successful results in children with diarrhea treated by rectal insufflation of the oxygen-ozone gas.

At the same ozone congress, I presented the results of my research with oxygen-ozone gas directly injected into the mammary carcinoma of the C3H/HeJ mice. This resulted in tumor death at the injection site with no apparent side effects. The control groups showed progressive cancer growth with no evidence of tumor death. The treated-healthy controls did not show side effects. All these findings were confirmed by histologic studies of Hematoxylin and Eosin (H&E) stained tissue sections and by electron microscopy. The H&E sections showed extensive coagulation necrosis and tumor cell death at the oxygen-ozone-treated site, while the untreated controls demonstrated no evidence of tumor death. Electron microscope studies of the oxygen-ozone-treated tumors demonstrated marked cellular disruption with alteration of the cells membranes, nuclei, and cytoplasms. No viral particles were found in the oxygen-ozone-treated areas, while the untreated controls have numerous viral particles and membrane budding.

Electron microscope studies of RBCs of the oxygen-ozone-treated tumors showed the RBC membranes to be free of immunocomplexes coating, while the RBCs of the nontreated human patients with breast cancer had extensive coating by immunocomplexes. The treated-healthy controls had no demonstrable changes at the injection site.

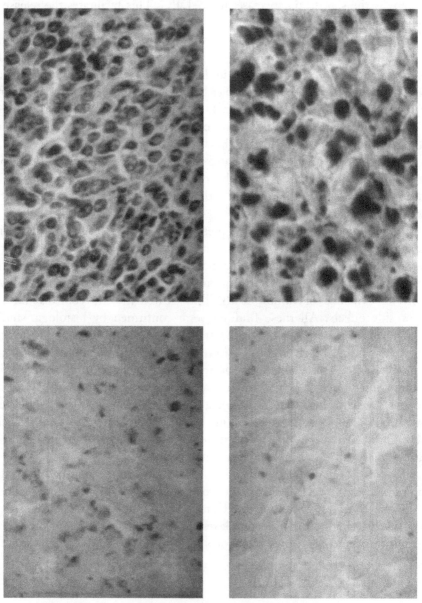

1 & 2 Photomicrograph of untreated mammary adenocarcinoma of the C3H/HeJ mouse (Magnifications: 10×50 and 10×100)

3 & 4 Photomicrographs of ozone, (O2/O3) treated adenocarcinoma of the C3H-HeJ mouse showing extensive tumor death and coagulation necrosis.

Examination of the treated and untreated bits of fresh tumor suspended in normal saline disclosed the presence of a few green granules (GG) or droplets in the cancer cell's cytoplasm. The GG appeared within minutes of observation by light microscopy and at room temperature. Upon further observation, the GG increased in size and in number until the whole cancer cell was occupied by them. Eventually, the cell burst, freeing the GG within the saline solution.

Effect of Ozone in Human Cancer Cells in the Laboratory

In 1980, Frederick Sweet et al. reported in science how the growth of human cancer cells in the lungs, breast, and uterus were "selectively inhibited in a dose-dependent manner by ozone." They concluded that "the mechanism for defense against ozone damage are impaired in human cancer cells." Healthy control cells were not affected by ozone.

Since cancer cells have an anaerobic metabolism and oxygen is not beneficial to its growth, it is easy to understand why ozone, an allotropic form of oxygen being more reactive than oxygen, cannot only inhibit cancer cell growth but also kills cancer cells.

Sweet's experiment supported my findings in the experimental animals with mammary carcinoma of the C3H/HeJ mice.

While my preliminary findings are encouraging, there is much work to be done. This form of experimental treatment cannot be used as the only means of cancer treatment, but in liaison with other treatments and with concomitant nutritional support and vitamin supplementation, especially antioxidants such as selenium, vitamins A, C, and E.

Findings in Human Cancers

Intrigued by the "green granules phenomenon" (GG) and being a pathologist able to obtain fresh cancer tissue, I examined every fresh tissue specimen obtained from the operating room—both cancerous and noncancerous, from then on.

I observed that when living human cancer cells were suspended in saline solution and were examined with the light microscope under high magnification (oil immersion 10×100), after few minutes, the GG appeared in the cancer cell's cytoplasm. These granules increased in size and in number until they occupied the whole cytoplasm, and then the cancer cell disintegrated, releasing the GG into the saline solution. What are these GG? Are the GG related to the amount of protein present in cancer tissue in the form of antibodies? Does protein-rich cancer tissue, when suspended in saline and under the influence of microscope light, release "coacervates" in the form of GG? Coacervates were described by

Oparin as water-dissolved proteins that become ionized or acquire an electrical charge. Once charged, they attract and bond water molecules, producing a shell. This mixture of salt and various organic molecules includes polypeptides, and nucleic acids may assemble new and complex molecular aggregates—"a stage of prebiochemical evolution," "coacervates" as suggested by Oparim. Do these "coacervates" containing hemoglobin pigment, as engulfed by the cancer cells, transmute the hemoglobin into chlorophyll pigment by a photochemical reaction when exposed to light? If not, then why the spontaneous appearance of the GG? Why green and not red, yellow, or brown? What are these GG? What is their significance? Are "coacervates" and GG one and the same?

Effect of Light on Cancer Cells

Examined bits of treated and untreated tumor controls, suspended in saline solution, under the light microscope, disclosed again the appearance of GG as previously observed in O_2-O_3-treated tumors. Thus, it appears that the GG were unrelated to the treatment, but definitely related to cancer since no GG were observed in saline suspended normal tissues.

The GG phenomenon could be reproduced in all cancers studied. These included cancer of the breast, stomach, colon, ovary, prostate, squamous carcinoma of the skin, and in one case of leiomyoma of the leg. However, a fresh bone marrow specimen from a case of chronic lymphocytic leukemia examined with the same technique showed no GG. No GG were observed in healthy or in noncancerous human tissues, but it could be found in every case of cancer examined.

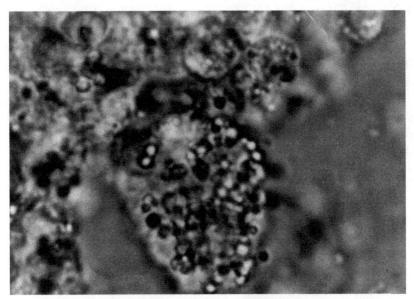

Saline-suspended cancer cell of the C3H/HeJ mouse distended
with green granules after light exposure

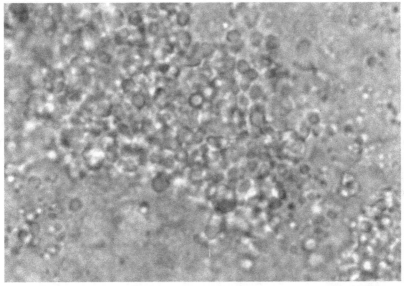

Within one hour of light exposure, the cell burst, freeing the green
granules into the saline solution.

Differences Between the Human and the Mice Green Granules

While the GG were observed in both in the mammary carcinoma of the C3H/HeH mice and in all cases of human cancers studied as previously listed, there were some differences.

The GG manifested readily in the mice's carcinoma. But in human cancers, the more immature or poorly differentiated the cancer is, the quicker was the appearance of the GG. Similar behavior was noted in other well-differentiated and slow-growing animal tumors. But in these cases, the GG were less numerous and it took longer to appear. Transplanted tumors did not develop GG too well either.

Benign tumors showed few or no green granules. The only normal cells to contain green granules were the macrophages from cancerous tissues and from inflammatory lesions. However, the GG found in these macrophages were uniformly larger than those observed in the cancer cells. Also to be noted is that the macrophages did not disintegrate as the cancer cells did when filled with the GG. The green color of the GG in the macrophages was less intense than the emerald green color observed in the cancer cell GG.

Characteristic of the Cancer Cell Green Granules

At first, the GG appeared as tiny specks in the cancer cell's cytoplasm, gradually increasing in number and in size to about 3mu. The cancer cell ruptured when filled with the GG. The freed GG appeared to have Brownian movements, and while some were budding, others coalesced. The GG were surrounded by a green-yellow halo resembling fluorescence.

For the GG to appear, there was a need for high light intensity in the microscope at standard room temperature. Lowering the temperature retarded or inhibited the appearance of the GG. There was light-dependency; control specimens placed in the dark for half an hour, then observed under the light microscope, failed to show GG. However, GG appeared in these specimens when observed for few minutes under the light.

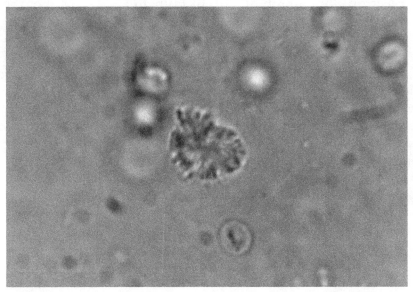

Bursting cancer cell after O$_2$-O$_3$ (oxygen-ozone) treatment

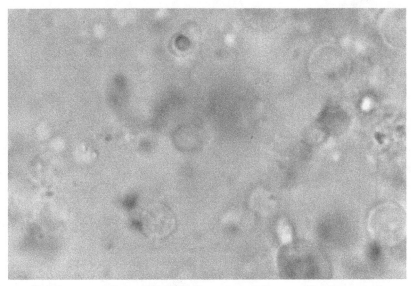

Dead cancer cells and few RBCs aspirated from an O$_2$-O$_3$-treated mammary adenocarcinoma of the C3H/HeJ mouse

Electron Photograph Studies of Human Cancers and of the O$_2$-O$_3$ Treated and Untreated Mammary Carcinoma of the C3H/HeJ Mouse

Investigation on the nature of the GG led me into electron photograph studies of the O$_2$-O$_3$-treated and untreated mammary carcinoma of the C3H/HeJ mouse. Electron photographic studies extended to several human cancers, including mammary carcinoma, melanoma, papillary carcinoma of the ovary, and of the globulin fraction of plasma from a patient with advanced metastatic mucus producing adenocarcinoma of the colon.

A most striking finding was a clear halo or area around the RBCs of the O$_2$-O$_3$-treated mouse tumor. The intravascular space was cleaner with much less immunocomplexes compared with the abundance of immunocomplexes intravascularly and coating the RBCs of the untreated human breast cancer. Compare the electron photographs in text.

Why the O$_2$-O$_3$-treated mouse tumor showed marked reduction of the immunocomplexes coating the RBCs and in the blood vessel lumen? Was the ozone treatment destroying the immunocomplexes and cleaning the blood?

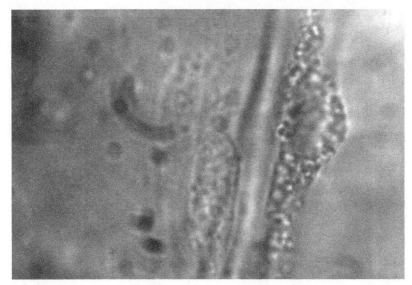

Human leiomyosarcoma cell distended with green granules after light exposure

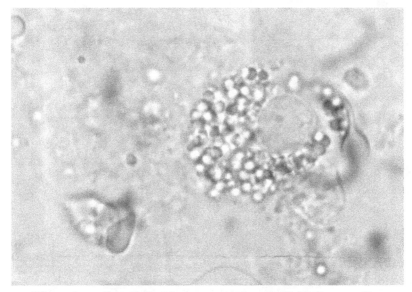

Macrophage distended with green granules after light exposure. But the macrophages did not burst as the cancer cells do.

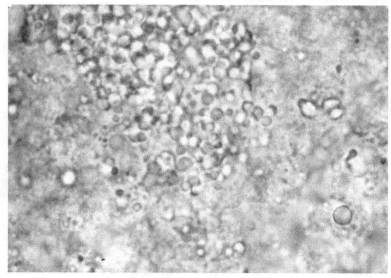

Cancer cells of the C3H/HeJ mouse distended with green granules after light exposure

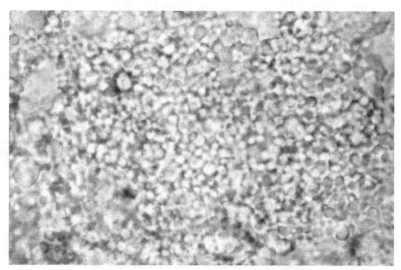

Numerous green granules (GG) in saline after cancer cells of the C3H/HeJ mouse were exposed to the light

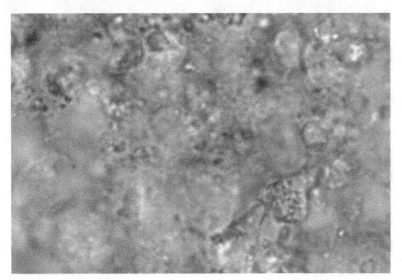

Human cancer cells with green granules after light exposure

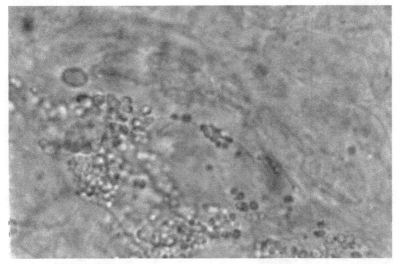

Human cancer cells from an adenocarcinoma of the breast containing green granules in their cytoplasm when exposed to the light while in saline solution

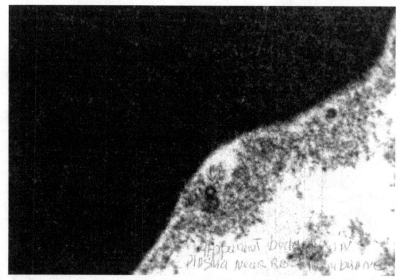

Untreated human blood from cancer of the breast, showing numerous immunecomplexes, coating the RBC surface and in the plasma

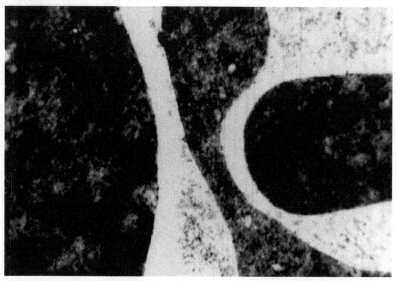

Ozone-treated mouse blood with adenocarcinoma of the mammary gland, with much less immunocomplexes in the plasma and almost none coating the red blood cells membrane

The immunocomplexes, by coating and plugging pores of the RBC and other tissue cell's membranes, inhibit the normal physiology of the cells; and thus, oxygenation of the tissues is impaired. If the RBCs cannot perform their physiologic needs, then their life span will be shortened, and the RBCs will more likely be phagocytized.

Thus far, I have been unable to identify the GG in the electron photographs. Perhaps this is due to inadequate light exposure of the tissues prior to processing. Another possibility is that the GG may be loose lipoproteins that might get lost during tissue processing.

Dr. Otto Rokitansky of Austria, at the Sixth Ozone World Congress, held in Washington DC, presented scanning electron microscope pictures of untreated and treated RBCs with ozone in a concentration of 20 μg/mL.

He pointed out how the ozone-treated RBCs did not aggregate in rouleaux formation as the untreated did. The freeing of the RBC cells facilitates the blood flow and the release of oxygen to the tissues. He found that ozone increased the elasticity of the RBCs' membranes, accelerated glucose metabolism, and increased the quantity of 2,3-DPG. The increased 2,3-DPG facilitates the release of oxygen.

Working with ozone, I have also found that the RBCs' elasticity and fluidity are increased with reduction or total elimination of rouleaux formation when using ozone concentrations from 20 to 35 μg/mL. Higher concentrations of ozone, ranging from 40 to 50 μg/mL, are likely to produce deformations of the RBCs with alteration of the cell membranes that could lead to hemolysis.

Ozone (O_3) is considered most helpful in all conditions requiring oxygenation. It is being used in other countries in cases of impaired circulation, allergies, hepatitis, hypercholesterolemia, in the treatment of cancer in combination with other therapies, in cases of gangrene, herpes, candidiasis, in skin ulcerations, and experimentally in acquired immune deficiency syndrome (AIDS).

Quantosomes in spinach chloroplast

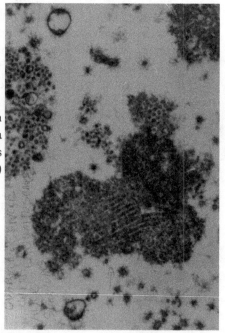

Electron photograph of human
ovarian papillary adenocarcinoma
with quantosome-like structures
(Magnification: x32,500)

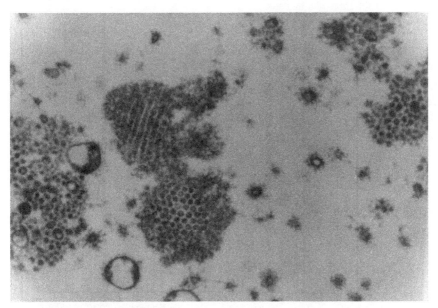

Electron photograph of quantosome-like particles in human ovarian cancer

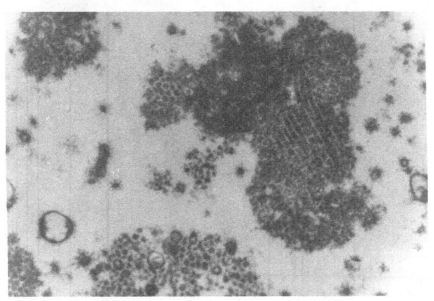

Higher magnification of the same photograph as above

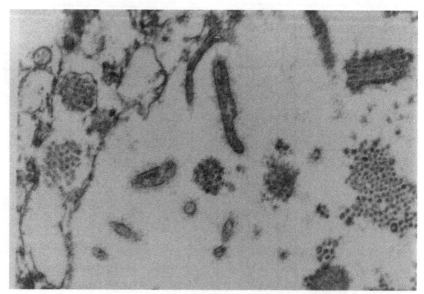

Electron photograph of human ovarian papillary carcinoma

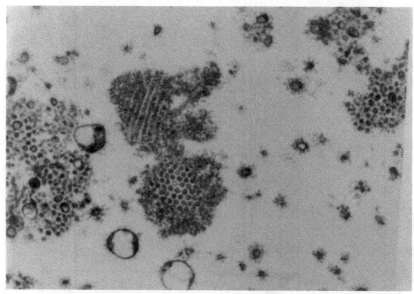

Electron photograph of human ovarian papillary carcinoma with quantosome-like particles. This is the only cancer with this particular finding.

Hemoglobin has four pyrroles and a central molecule of iron, while chlorophyll has magnesium at its center. Is it possible for the cancer cell to transmute the central iron molecule from the hemoglobin to magnesium and thus produce a primitive form of chlorophyll when cancer cells are exposed to the proper light? Much research is needed before this can be answered.

Under light exposure, there is photooxidation of the cancer cell, and if the following phenomenon occurs, it could explain the formation of chlorophyll and the release of active oxygen (O_3), with subsequent destruction of the cancer cells. If light-exposed cancer cells in saline solution can transmute iron (Fe++) of the hemoglobin molecule obtained from the engulfed RBCs to magnesium (Mg++), and the following reaction takes place:

$$Fe++(56) - S(32) = Mg(24) + O_2(32)$$

Then under proper circumstances, it is possible that the cancer cells may produce a very primitive form of chlorophyll, thus accounting for the green granules (GG) and for the oxygen release (active oxygen, O_3) that kills the cancer cells freeing the GG.

Other researchers, such as Weis in 1942, pointed out that "in certain molecular complexes, an electron can go spontaneously from one molecule—the donor to another—the acceptor, a reaction termed 'change transfer'." Something similar occurs with the enzyme glycoxalase for the conversion of alphaketoaldehydes to unreactive oxyacids. This indicates the participation of oxygen molecules. Similar mechanism is observed with the quinones. The quinones act as strong oxidizing agents.

The oxidative action of the quinones is observed in the color changes occurring in areas of plant damage. Similarly, the bacteria-killing effect of the quinones is due to the release of phenol oxidase, again an oxidation phenomenon. Albert Szent-Gyorgi mentioned at the International Symposium on Cancer Research in 1984, "Once a cell loses the ability to bind its own glycoxalase, it will go on endless multiplication behaving like a cancer cell." This emphasizes the importance of oxidation in the maintenance of the cell's health. If oxidation is reduced, accumulation of cellular wastes will occur, and aging and disease will follow. Cancer cells have lost the oxidative mechanism necessary for the maintenance of physiology of healthy cell.

Szent-Gyorgi, who has worked on biological oxidation mechanisms, suggested in 1941 that within the living systems there is a semi-conduction phenomenon. He postulated that macromolecules such as proteins are organized to function as a crystalline lattice.

In 1952, March and Beams reported a series of experiments on plenaria, a simple flat worm with a primitive nervous system. Electrical measurements demonstrated a simple head-tail dipole field. When the worm was cut transversally into various segments, all regenerated into a complete new organisms. Furthermore, the regenerated parts had the same original head-tail orientation as the original. March et al. proposed that the original electrical vector persisted in the segments, thus providing information for regeneration. With further experimentation, they were able to produce heads at both ends of the segments, but with increased electrical impulse, the expected head-tail reversal occurred. This gives some inkling of the marked influence that the environment has on organisms.

Rapid growing tissues are electronegative in polarity. This fact is more prominent in tumors. Humprey and Seal applied copper or zinc anodes over tumor implants in rats. The mean control volume was seven times greater than the test animals, and while the controls died by the thirty-first day, seven of the eighteen treated animals survived over a year after the treatment.

Szent-Gyorgi's concept is that cancer-causing agents produce their effect by a combination of the steric organization and their capacity for electron transfer. This was proven by Huggins and Yang in 1962 with their experiments on the induction and extinction of mammary cancer.

The principle has been applied therapeutically by Dr. C. Andrew Basset of Columbia University, New York to orthopedic cases with non-union of long-bone fractures.

Free Radicals, Oxygen, and Ozone

Free radicals are the by-product of chemical reactions in the body. If electrons charged with energy are not neutralized, it can promote cancer development. Free radical electrons charged with energy have neutron displaced out of an atom's orbit. The free radical energy is transferred to many substances producing damage.

Oxygen is essential for life, but single oxygen has high energy, and if unstable, it can be damaging to tissues. It can be damaging or helpful; depending on the circumstances, however. The active oxygen is utilized by the macrophages to destroy toxins, bacteria, or viruses. Because of its high reactivity, single oxygen has a short life span. Ozone (O_3) reacts with molecules in the body, and it stimulates the production of peroxides which helps neutralize cell wastes.

Opposite to free radicals, vitamin C, vitamin E, and selenium are free radical scavengers that help neutralize free radicals.

CHAPTER VIII

Protein Molecules
Tridimensional Confirmation

By its complex structure, proteins represent the greatest structural organization within a particular molecule. The tridimensional structure of proteins was discovered by Kendrew and Peruts by using x-ray diffraction. Their discovery, that the myoglobulin of the sperm whale has a tridimensional organization, won them the Nobel Prize in 1965.

The arrangement of the amino acids in the stereoscopic protein molecule is of the utmost importance. Amino acids, the building blocks of proteins, can be hydrophobic or hydrophylic. The hydrophylic amino acids are normally situated at the periphery of the protein molecule where interactions with water occur. The hydrophobic amino acids are located on the inside of the protein molecule, thus protected from water.

Normal positioning of the amino acids is indispensable for the proper interchange and physiology. Its significance is reflected in sickle cell anemia, in which the abnormal hemoglobin has the hydrophylic glutamic acid replacing the hydrophobic valine found in normal hemoglobin.

The amino acid replacement has altered the hemoglobin molecule. The altered hemoglobin, if deprived of oxygen, becomes insoluble and precipitates in the form of crystals in the red blood cells, thus giving the sickle cell appearance. Because of the new altered form, RBCs tend to aggregate, thus inhibiting even more the oxygen exchange. With the reduction of oxygen transport, there is progressive tissue hypoxia and anemia.

Proteins are very large molecules, some having molecular weight of few millions. Variations in amino acids give protein its different physical and chemical properties, and these will reflect in the various functions.

Changes in a single amino acid in the hemoglobin alter not only the morphology, but also its physiology. Alterations of other molecules may have a dramatic impact in the body's physiology; some alterations may be incompatible with life.

Cell Transformation, Molecular Changes at the Cell Surface

Cancer cells have lost the cellular affinity found in normal cells. If skin cancer cells are mixed with normal kidney cells, there is an even intermingling of the two cell types. In mixing normal kidney cells with normal liver cells, the cells from each particular organ aggregated and stayed together but did not mix with the other organ cells.

In my electron photograph studies of cancer tissue, I have observed a thick layer of electron-dense particles coating the cancer cell plasma membrane and coating the adjacent noncancerous cells as well. Is this cellular coating dulling the cell membrane sensors and thus facilitating the intermingling of normal and cancer cells, as well as permitting cancer infiltration? Does this coat of cancer antigen and immunocomplexes inhibit the body from rejecting the cancerous cells?

Not only there are alterations in cancer cells' glycoprotein membranes, but also secretion of proteolytic enzymes, which facilitate infiltration in most cancer cells.

Antibody Composition

Cancer cells have large nuclei and small cytoplasms. Nucleotides are derived from amino acids—the building blocks of proteins. In a cell's cytoplasm, RNA molecules in the ribosomes are responsible for the amino acids in the proper sequence to form proteins. How can cancer cells be able to perform this function with such scanty cytoplasm where the ribosomal DNA is located?

It seems that the protein has to be readily available to the cancer cell from outside, since the cancer cell lacks the machinery available to manufacture it as normal cells do.

For its nutrition and for continuous cell division, cancer cells use protein and antibodies produced by the plasma cells. Therefore, cancer cells depend upon other cells for its nutritional needs.

Nucleotides can be incorporated into DNA chains by enzymatic reactions during repair processes. Is it possible for the same repair process to continuously occur in cancer cells in an effort to reach intracellular homeostasis?

Antibodies or immuneglobulins are complex protein molecules that combine with their specific antigen in a "lock and key" fashion. Five different immunoglobulins have been described in man: IgG, IgM, IgA, IgD, and IgE. Of all the immunoglobulins, IgG, the smallest, can cross the placenta.

Antibodies are produced against proteins of different kinds including bacteria, viruses, parasites, and fungi. There are receptors for IgG on the plasma membrane of human monocytes and in some lymphocytes. IgG is found in the intravascular spaces.

The largest of the immunoglobulins, IgM, is the first to appear after an antigenic response, and it is followed by IgG. IgM is found intravascularly, and when its concentration is increased, it can agglutinate RBCs and bacteria.

Other immunoglobulins, such as IgE, are associated with skin allergic reactions; and IgA is found in the excretory system, respiratory, gastrointestinal, and genitourinary tracts.

Composition of the Immunoglobulins

Immunoglobulins are composed of a basic unit of two large or heavy chains and two small or light chains united by disulfide bonds. The heavy chains are centrally placed parallel to each other and joined by disulfide bonds.

The light chains are parallel to the heavy chains and are joined by disulfide bonds also. By using proteolitic enzymes, specific fragments of the immunoglobulin (antibody), have been identified. The fragments vary in functions and in some of the amino acids' composition.

Specificity of the Antibodies

Antibodies are highly specific. This specificity depends on the sequence of amino acids. Each antibody fits its antigenic site, as the key fits its lock. Since antibodies are produced by the plasma cells in response to antigen stimulation, plasma cells must recognize and replicate a mirror image of the antigenic site in order for the antibodies to be specific.

Is there a particular amino acid or sequence of amino acids that are more immunogenic than others? If so, which are those? Where are they situated in the antigenic molecule? Does the enhancement of antigenicity depend not only on the nature of the amino acids present, but also in how the amino acids are arranged?

Each antibody has a constant and a variable region. The amino acid, terminal of the heavy and light chains, is the antibody-active or antigen-binding site. This corresponds to the variable region; the constant region (constant amino acids sequence) contains the carboxyl terminal.

Susuki and Deutcsh reported on the average amino acid composition of six human yM immunoglobulins, and Kochwa et al. compared it with the IgE myeloma protein. It was found "that the main difference between IgE and IgM was a high cystine and methionine content of this protein."

There are antibodies specific for either the light or heavy chain of the antigen. The antigen binding site of the antibody is located in the NH_2 terminal end of the variable portion of the immunoglobulin. It represents about 1 percent of the total immunoglobulin molecule.

The electrical charge of the antigenic site must be compatible with the antibody's variable region NH_2 terminus. Therefore, the amino acid sequence and relationship to one another must be of the utmost importance, not only in immunogenic potential, but in specificity as well.

Edelman in 1959 published his findings of the multichain structure of the immunoglobulins. On stereoscopic or tridimensional representation of the immunoglobulin molecule, there is a grove formation between the variable regions of the light and heavy chains. It is at this level where the specificity of the antigenic determinant and the site of attachment are found. This is also the site of the hypervariable region.

Before an antibody is produced, it needs an antigenic stimulant. This can be in the form of a foreign protein, bacteria, or virus. The antigenic substance would normally be engulfed by the macrophages, which are part of the reticuloendothelial system (RES). By doing so, the macrophage becomes sensitized. But there are no obvious clinical manifestations on the first contact with the foreign antigenic substance. Only with subsequent stimulations of the same type of antigen may clinical manifestations occur.

Thus, the sensitized macrophages will transform into lymphocytes that subsequently will transform into specific antibody-producing plasma cells once the second and subsequent stimulations occur.

For example, diabetics used to receive insulin made from beef or sheep for many years; then the patients started to develop resistance to it with antibody production. By changing to pig insulin, the treatment can be continued. The difference between the two sources of insulin lies in the sequence of three amino acid units in one segment. It is at this level where the antigenicity resides.

To explain the great reactivity of the immune system, Burnett suggested that an infinite number of silent genes must be available in the chromosomes for the possible infinite stimulants.

By measuring DNA synthesis by autoradiography, Burnett found that young plasma blasts divide once every ten hours. According to him, it appears that "starting with a single plasma blast, there are typically nine successive divisions producing a clone or colony of cells before division stops."

With the iodine-125-labeled antigen, Burnett noticed that "the antigen was very efficiently gobbled up by the large scavenger cells or macrophages. The macrophages deep within the lymph nodes proved to be loaded with the antigen."

Is it possible that the primitive totipotential macrophage, by gobbling up antigenic molecules, become primed? Later on, primed macrophage could develop into plasma cells with the ability to produce specific antibodies in the form of a mirror image of the priming antigen, therefore assuring a perfect-fit "lock and key" match.

Protein molecules may act as switches by changing their shapes. This may be influenced by the changes in the pH, electric charges, and temperature. Such alterations, therefore, can facilitate abnormal changes in the cellular behavior. Such alterations can be observed in autoimmune diseases.

T cells react when the cell receptor identifies foreign antigen. The antigen is associated with a histocompatible molecule whereby there is recognition of self and nonself.

Self-tolerance or discrimination between self and nonself may be true to a point. Once a specific organ has been damaged at the cellular level, whereby ribosomal DNA and other intracellular organelles are exposed to the surface membrane of other intact surfaces, such as macrophages (RES), sensitization is prone to occur. Each cell system has its own specific proteins and enzymes that are foreign or extrinsic to other organ systems. Therefore, it seems logical that an immune response be elicited when there is extracellular leakage in the cell's content.

With repeated cell damage and leakage, further sensitization and immune reaction could occur, eventually developing into one of the many autoimmune or degenerative diseases. The causes of which are unexplainable at the moment.

Since macrophages are stimulated and attracted to injured sites while collecting cellular debris, macrophages could become sensitized; and thus, maturing plasma cells are able to produce specific antibodies. Upon further stimulation, the sensitized mature plasma cells will produce enough tissue-specific antibodies that will eventually lead to chronic degenerative diseases with progressive clinical manifestations. The interval between the initial stimulus and clinical symptoms can vary from days to years (e.g., thyroiditis, hepatitis, myositis, arthritis, and others).

According to Jerne, each plasma cell "must transcribe its antibody genes into 20,000 messenger-RNA molecules that serve 200,000 ribosomes, enabling the cell to produce and secrete 2,000 identical antibodies per second." With such an antibody-producing capability in each plasma cell, it is easy to understand its pathogenic potential when its target is the body's own tissues.

If the reticuloendothelial system (RES, macrophages) in cancer patients reacts in a similar manner to the cancer antigen/s by producing an exhausting and continuous amount of antibodies, it is easy to understand why cancer patients are susceptible to all kinds of infections. Their immune system is so saturated and sensitized to the specific cancer antigen/s that there are no immunoblasts with free and available antigenic site able to respond to a different antigenic stimulus. The cancer patient's immune system is oversaturated with the cancer's antigen. Thus, there is no defense against exposure to bacteria, fungi, or viruses.

The cancer patient is unable to defend itself in spite of an overactive immune system, a system saturated with the cancer antigen. As the cancer progresses and spreads, any remaining immune defense is completely lost. With continuation of the cancer's mass growth, there is a proportional increase in the amount of cancer wastes or antigen/s produced. With the progression of the disease and toward its end-stage, there is a greater predisposition to all kind of infections.

Immune Defense System

The immune system is composed of B lymphocytes (bursa-derived), T lymphocytes (thymus-derived), and the macrophages (RES). Based on microscopic studies of lymph nodes, connective tissues and organ tissues including intestinal, spleen liver, and thymus, it appeared as if as if the cells representing the immune system are all derived from the reticuloendothelial system within the particular organ, regulated by the thymus, and/or bursa as need be.

The RES of a particular organ may be already primed to produce differentiation into the different immunological components—B or T lymphocytes and macrophages. The macrophages, being the less differentiated, are more likely to have totipotential ability.

Jerne reported that "more than 10^{10} new lymphocytes arise in the thymus every day. The majority of these cells are killed in the thymus, or immediately after they leave it." If this is so, where do the tissue lyphocytes come from? They will have to be originated or derived from the tissue macrophages in situ, after being primed by some thymic or bursa hormone.

There is a close relationship between the B lymphocytes and the T lymphocytes. If one is deficient, the other cannot function effectively.

Cultures of spleen lymphocytes (B lymphocytes), together with an antigenic substance, fail to produce antibody unless T lymphocytes are added to the culture. Then B lymphocytes start to produce antibodies against the antigen.

It is interesting to note that normal and healthy T lymphocytes and B lymphocytes cannot be cultures as yet. While B lymphocytes infected by the Epstein-Barr virus will produce monoclonal cell lines, T cell lines from malignant conditions are nor suitable for unraveling the normal physiology of the T cell, or for the identification of the T cell–specific receptors.

Allergy, Vaccine, and Immunity in the Pathogenesis of Disease

Allergic reactions manifest in the skin in various forms such as edema, redness, itching, scaling, blisters, hives, and others. These manifestations give clues to the ravaging effect produced by the immune response affecting the internal organs. The significance and the degree of its damage will go unrecognized if clinical symptoms are not obvious. Thus, sensitization and the damage continue silently until tissue or organ damage is severe enough to become obvious. By then, the disease process is well established and manifests itself by affecting a particular organ or system with a disease to which the individual may be genetically disease prone to. Such may be the case in diabetes, rheumathoid arthritis, artheriosclerosis, collagen diseases, multiplesclerosis, and others, including aging and cancer.

With the above in mind, it seems reasonable to limit vaccination or any kind of immunization to the most dangerous and life-threatening situations. Routine vaccination for the prevention of less threatening conditions should not be mandatory, but instead proper nutrition and exercise must be encouraged as a preventive measure.

Diseases appear when the body is polluted by toxic materials and wastes, thus creating the proper environment for infections and other diseases to develop. Diseases manifest as an effort of the body to get rid of undesirable elements. The attempted eliminations are manifested as fever, diarrhea, vomitus, or other body manifestations.

With proper nutrition, fresh food, free of pollutants such as artificial coloring or flavoring, insecticides, and by daily exercises, and developing peace of mind, most diseases can be prevented.

Vaccination may be responsible for the initial triggering or sensitizing element, which years later will manifest in the form of chronic or degenerative disease. The disease may affect a particular organ or system according to the individual predisposition.

Dr. Robert W. Simpson while addressing the American Cancer Society Seminar for Writers noted that "immunization programs against flu, measles, mumps, and polio may actually be seeding humans with RNA to form pro-viruses which will then become latent cells . . . some of these latent pro-viruses could be molecules in search of diseases which under proper conditions become activated and cause a variety of diseases . . . including rheumathoid arthritis, multiple sclerosis, lupus erythematosus, Parkinson's disease, and perhaps cancer."

Ida Honorot and E. McBean, in their book *Vaccination the Silent Killer*, reported on Dr. Simpsom's response to her inquiry on the swine flu vaccine. His reply being "while the occurrence of swine flu next year as a major pandemic strain is highly questionable, public health authorities have been placed in a position whereby they have no other recourse, but to proceed with a large scale immunization."

In 1959, still a Cuban citizen, while returning from a two-week vacation in Cuba, and being five months pregnant, I was forced to be vaccinated for smallpox upon entry back into the United States in spite of no epidemic or exposure. All my pleading was to no avail. The officer was not allowing my entry at the border unless I was vaccinated in spite of my pregnancy. I just had left United States for two weeks after living in the country for five consecutive years during my internship and my pathology specialty training. Interestingly enough, my husband, an American citizen, traveling with me was not required to be vaccinated.

My only child, a daughter, thanks to God, was born healthy, but years later we found out that there was damage to one of her auditory nerves. Was this nerve damage vaccine related?

Dr. Jonas Salk and Darrell Salk reported in science, March 4, 1977, "Live virus vaccines against influenza and paralytic poliomyelitis may in each instance produce the disease it intends to prevent . . . The live virus vaccine against measles and mumps may produce such side effects as encephalitis (brain damage) and kill virus vaccines against measles, and the respiratory syncitial virus have caused undesirable hypersensitivity reactions in individuals subsequently exposed to natural infections."

In February 1977, HEW Secretary Joseph Caliano stated, continues Honorof, "The swine vaccine cannot be given legally, unless those receiving it sign a 'consent' form."

Vaccines are usually prepared with the attenuated or dead virus or bacteria, with added egg protein, formalin, and other preservatives. Some people may be allergic to egg protein and to formalin. Formalin is a water solution of formaldehyde. This has been proven to be not only toxic, but carcinogenic, when injected under the skin of rats.

During immunization, various reactions may occur. Although the risk of serious injury from certain vaccines for childhood diseases is rare, the incident of convulsions in diphtheria immunization is one in a million.

Data from the NIH on October 1976 and January 20–21, 1977, disclosed that the first dosage of swine vaccine were given on October 1 and by December 1. There were over 40 million people vaccinated all under the National Influenza Immunization Program. Within two weeks, by mid-December, the surveillance system within the immunization program detected "an increased incidence of Guillan-Barre syndrome among the vacinated." While a moratorium was placed on the influenza vaccination program, preliminary statistics showed that "the risk of Guillan-Barre was approximately 10 times greater in the vaccinated than in the non-vaccinated." Worldwide surveillance under the World Health Organization revealed no swinelike viruses occurring in man elsewhere in the world.

Family Practice News in its December 1–14, 1984, issue on page 22 reported on the disagreement over the benefits of the pertussis vaccine. In countries such as Japan and Great Britain, "the public has not been convinced of the benefits of immunization" and in "West Germany and Sweden, the toxicity of the vaccines has been judged to outweigh their benefits and they are recommended only for high risk groups."

In the same article, the effectiveness of the vaccines is questioned, and the mortality rate in "France, Britain, and West Germany are almost identical, despite immunizations rates of 95 percent, 40 percent and 10 percent," Dr. T Rollfors notes.

Allergic Manifestations

Diseases such as asthma, hay fever, urticaria, and job related allergies are manifestations of an immediate type of hypersensitivity reaction from individuals to a variety of allergens. IgE antibodies are found in the patient sera. These antibodies attach to the mast cells and produce degranulation of these cells, and precipitating the release of histamine an anaphylaxis mediator.

Membrane Surface Receptors

The glycoproteins of the cell membrane appear to be the receptor or recognition site for antigens (hormones, viruses, etc.). Some glycoproteins are heterogeneous in their carbohydrate component. There is supporting evidence that this component may be able to change under different conditions while the polypeptide remains unchanged.

Buck, Glick, and Warren have demonstrated that normal and malignant cells have a different protein-bound carbohydrate groups. These bound carbohydrate groups are influenced by their environment in cell cultures, such as concentration of the serum and the type of buffer as demonstrated by Megaw and Johnson.

The immunologic response of the mammals becomes activated when the lymphoid tissue of the gastrointestinal tract is stimulated by nutrients' antigenic substances and to the intestinal flora. It has been demonstrated that the payer patches of the germfree rats are composed of "small lymphocytes with rudimentary germinal center," while the conventionally fed rats have "large germinal center with a cluster of basophylic lymphoblasts." The centers and the corona contained large amounts of macrophages. Traskalova-Hogenova et al.'s findings show that the payer's patches contain cells producing immunoglobulins and that "these cells differentiated in situ into antibody-forming cells."

These findings support the view that lymphocytes and plasma cells can originate in situ from cells of the RES system (macrophages) or connective tissue cells.

The mucosa of the gastrointestinal tract, urinary tract, and others protect the internal organs from the outside. Certain bacteria have specific preference for mucosal surface, such as the gram negative E. coli, Klebsiella, Proteous mirabilis, and others for the urinary tract. S. Eden et al. suggest that there is an adhesive factor that predisposes the attachment of bacteria to a specific spithelium.

The bacteria bind to the glycolipid binding sites by fimbriae (pili). Thus, by this local attachment, focal irritation and infection may initiate an immune response to the bacteria-glycolipids that can lead to disease.

Chapter IX

The Immunologic Basis of Diseases

Over seventy years ago, Dr. Clemens von Pirquet suggested that the body's response to an antigen may be toxic to the body as he observed in serum sickness. This disease is produced by the injection of foreign blood serum to patients already containing antibodies in their blood against the foreign serum protein.

Rosenberg and Farber at the NIH found that when lymphocytes from animals immunized with herpes virus (HSV) were incubated in a test tube with HSV antigen, the antigen turned on the lymphocytes to replicate the DNA and to divide. "This reaction began within hours after the exposure to the antigen, and was quite specific: they did not react to all the antigens of other viruses."

A virus researcher also at the NIH, Wallace P. Rowe in 1950s proved Von Pirquet's hypothesis while studying the pathologic changes produced by the virus that causes lymphocytic choriomeningitis (LCM). He noted that the virus-infected mice showed no signs of illness, although there was extensive proliferation of the virus. "On the sixth day, he noticed that after the mice started to produce an immune response to the virus, the mice developed meningitis and died."

It appears, therefore, that the virus itself does not directly produce disease; but instead, it is the immune's response to the virus. The antibodies then are the direct cause of the pathological process.

Subsequently, Rowe did an experiment where test mice were irradiated to destroy its immune system and a control group where the mice were not irradiated. Both groups were inoculated with LCM virus. He found that while the virus replicated in the irradiated mice, these mice did not develop meningitis. The control group (not irradiated) also showed viral replication, but they died. In this later case, the immune system was intact and reacted to the virus with an immune response that killed the mice. The irradiated mice that inhibited the immune system did not develop the disease.

A group of investigators from Johns Hopkins suppressed the immune system with drugs and then injected all the mice with the LCM virus. The animals were divided into three groups. The first group was treated with anti-CLM antibody, the second group was given anti-LCM lymphocytes, and the third group was treated with normal lymphocytes. "The animals receiving the antibody or the normal lymphocytes remained well, but those given the immune lymphocytes developed the symptoms of LCM disease and died."

The above experiments clearly prove that the virus is not directly responsible for the disease, but rather the immune response to the virus's antigen/s. The virus's antigen/s stimulates the B lymphocytes and plasma cells to produce specific antibodies. Therefore, antibody—as its name defines is anti, or against, and body, equals against the body—is the direct cause of the disease.

Infection of cells with certain viruses stimulates the virus-infected cells to produce viral antigens that are secreted by the infected cells' plasma membrane. The secreted viral antigens stimulate the B lymphocytes to produce plasma cells which in turn will produce viral-antigen-specific antibodies.

The viral-antigen-specific antibodies will attack the viral antigenic site of the virus-infected cell plasma membrane. This will block the membrane pores and will interfere with the cell's normal physiology and nutrition. Thus, a cell so blocked by antibodies is condemned to die.

The severity of the situation depends upon the importance of the function of the cell affected. Combination of antigens with antibodies form masses of immunocomplexes that can further inhibit the intracellular and intercellular nutrients and wastes exchanges by reducing the blood flow of tiny capillaries and by rouleaux formation of the antigen-antibody coated RBCs.

Chronic viral infections have characteristic viral-antibody complexes as observed in glomerulonephritis. Oldstone and Dixon demonstrated that LCM virus exists in the blood of the chronically infected animal as an infectious virus-antibody complex, and that the kidney contained large amounts of the LCM antigen, anti-LCM antibody, and complement.

Arthritis, diabetes, poststreptococcal glomerulonephritis, rheumathoid arthritis, viral hepatitis, and many other diseases are considered of an autoimmune nature.

Immune complexes have been demonstrated with immunofluorescent techniques and other methods.

Collagen diseases and mixed connective tissue disease can manifest as lupus erythematosus, scleroderma, Raynaud's phenomenon, and polymyositis.

These diseases may progress to the more advanced stage of systemic sclerosis. Raynaud's phenomenon is characterized by thickening of the blood vessel's walls with involvement of the intima. This phenomenon is seen in 95 percent of the sclerotic patients. Dr. Richard Stern, in the October 1984 issue of *Managing Pain and Presenting Symptoms* stated, "vascular sclerosis in the kidneys eventually leads to malignant hypertension, a leading cause of death in sclerosis patients. All these diseases have an immunologic background with extensive deposits of the immunocomplexes in the connective tissue slowly smothering the connective tissue and depriving it of the needed blood and nutrients."

It would be interesting to find out how many and what kind of vaccines patients with chronic degenerative diseases such as lupus, scleroderma, polymyositis, arthritis, and others have had, and compare it with the incidence of these diseases in the nonvaccinated population.

Viral Antibodies Associated With Malignancy

Nasopharyngeal carcinoma (NPC) has higher incidence in Chinese from Canton province compared with the incidence in the rest of the world population. Patients with NPC have high titer of antibodies against various Epstein-Barr virus (EBV) coded antigens.

The EBV virus was found by Epstein and colleagues in London while studying the Burkitt's lymphoma by electron microscopy. This EBV herpes virus was named after its discoverers, and it was found to give persistent viral markers to tumor cells, and was therefore considered oncogenic. Human or Simian B lymphocytes can be immortalized in vitro with the EBV virus. The EBV can induce lymphomas and reticulum cell sarcomas in the new world primates. Kurstack and Kurstack noted that "EBV transforming or immortalizing capacity is specific," but it can be neutralized by human sera containing antibodies against EBV.

Cytomegalic viruses (CMV), a group of viruses within the herpes virus family, have been described in 1904 by Jesionek and Kiolemenoglou, and also by Ribbert. It produces the "cytomegalic inclusion disease" in humans. The virus is found in the blood, urine, saliva, human milk, and semen.

The CMV is implicated in the pathogenesis of cervical cancer, congenital defects, mental retardation, prematurity, intrauterine death, interstitial pneumonia in organ-transplantation patients, and as the cause of hemolysis and autoimmune problems in some hemolytic anemias.

Various adenovirus types have been reported to be oncogenic to laboratory animals such as mice and hamsters. While most of the tumors produced are undifferentiated sarcomas, some may resemble lymphomas.

Certain human and animal adenoviruses can transform rats, hamsters, and rabbit cells in vitro, whether or not it has oncogenicity in vivo. It is interesting to note that infectious viruses cannot be detected in transformed cells in vitro or in vivo.

The Epstein-Barr virus is associated with infectious mononucleosis, Burkitt's lymphoma and nasophryngeal carcinoma. Greaves et al. in 1975 demonstrated that the B lymphocytes are the target cells for the virus (EBV). The EBV can transform normal lymphocytes into immortal cells in vitro. These transformed cells can be identified by their expression of multiple Epstein-Barr virus-specific nuclear antigen.

Few of the tests used for the detection of the CMV are immunofluorescence, complement fixation and neutralization, immunoperoxidase, and hemaglutination.

Human Tumor Viruses

While various animal oncogenic viruses can be easily identified within the tumors, this is not the case in humans. In the mammary carcinoma of the mice induced by the B-RNA virus (Bittner's particles), budding viral particles can easily be identified by electron microscope. Other RNA viruses produce lymphoid tumors of domestic fowl and kidney tumors of frogs.

These are RNA viruses (oncornaviruses) that utilize the host cell DNA to transcribe their single-stranded RNA. It is done by utilizing an enzyme, RNA-dependent DNA polymerase present in the core of the virions as described by Temin and Mitzutani in 1970, and also by Baltimore in 1970. This enzyme also called reverse transcriptase (RT or RDDP) was discovered simultaneously by Temin and Mitzutani in chicken sarcoma virus and by Baltimore in the Rauscher mouse leukemia virus. The reverse transcriptase enzyme characterizes the retroviruses group.

Like all polymerases, reverse transcriptase (RT) under the direction of an RNA template, makes DNA by adding deoxyribonucleotide triphosphates to each other in the direction 5'—>3'. It requires Mg^{2+} and Mn^{2+} for this reaction to occur.

Because of the presence of viral particles in animal tumor tissues, and in leukemic chickens, and in the milk of mice with mammary cancer, extensive work has been done in human trying to find viral elements.

Particles resembling B virus have been found in biopsy of human breast cancer. Similar elements have been found in human milk. Viral elements a have been found in blast cells of two patients with Chédiack-Higashi syndrome. Similar viruslike particles have been observed in biopsies of human sarcomas, bone tumors, and cancer of the prostate.

Two types of C virus were first isolated from human cell cultures. The ESP-1 virus was isolated from cells of pleural effusion from a young patient with Burkitt's lymphoma. The other virus RD-114 was isolated from cells of tissue culture of a rabdomyosarcoma as reported by Kurstack and Kurstack.

Recent reports reveal that cancers of viral and nonviral nature may be related to the activation or deactivation of similar cellular genes. These silent or dormant pro-oncogenes, present in normal cellular genes, can transform when infected by a virus. While the cancer cells transforming normal genes counterpart are considered to be originated by an unknown alteration of the normal gene. Of about fifteen viral pro-oncogenes (onc genes), two sarcoma related genes resemble human cancer cells oncogenes.

Viral Oncogenesis

Presently, there are two concepts of oncogenesis. One, the provirus theory of Temin proposed in 1964. His theory is that the RNA virus inserts its genetic information into the genome of the infested cells, and by means of the reverse transcriptase, the host DNA replication of the virus occurs.

Huebner and Tadaro in 1969 and Tadaro and Huebner in 1972, hypothesized that animal cells may carry viral genes. A portion of this gene may be oncogenic and the stimulus of various factors such as irradiation, autoantibodies, or other viruses. This gene can be activated, thus resulting in cell transformation. Probably a combination of the two hypotheses may be closer to the facts.

Immune Response in Tumor-Bearing Host

Yasushi Ono et al. in 1974 reported that "antigen-primed macrophages from normal mice failed to transmit antigen information to B and T cells in tumor-bearing mice." They concluded that the "transmission of antigen information from macrophages to B and T cells or subsequent early steps in antibody formation was suppressed in tumor-bearing mice."

I propose that the B and T cells from the cancerous animals were already primed by the cancer antigen and therefore committed. Further efforts to prime them would be useless, and therefore, sensitization and antibody production to any other but the cancer antigen would not be possible.

T Cell in Cancer

In patients with terminal cancer, the tissue's immune response is markedly impaired as observed in the decreased tuberculin sensitivity. Orita and coworkers found that the decrease was not dependent on the tumor cell count, but rather on the decline in function.

It seems logical that if the T cells are continuously dividing in an effort to protect the body against the cancer, they will eventually reach their fiftieth division; and thus, with an increased percentage of aging T cells, their competence could decline—they may die or transform. Another concomitant possibility is that the T cell's reactivity is impaired or inhibited by the cancer antigen.

Since the humoral antibodies do not contribute (B-cells) to the tissue's immune defense against cancer, the body is helpless against it, unless the T cells are responding properly.

I suggest that the way T cells balance the immune system is by producing a very active form of oxygen in the form of ozone (O_3). The ozone quickly neutralizes or destroys antibodies, toxins, bacteria, or viruses; thus, cellular balance is restored and disease is inhibited.

The recognition of the self and nonself depends not only on the reactivity of the T cells, but also on the integrity of the self (tissues). If the plasma membrane is damaged by necrosis, trauma, surgery, radiation, or chemicals, cellular organelles or fragments are exposed to the extracellular system. If the amount of damage is sufficient enough, with adequate leakage of the sensitizing intracellular substances, then it is possible that an autovaccine effect or autoimmune response will occur.

The autoimmune response may be in direct relationship with the amount of the tissue damage and with the degree of the tissue specialization. The greater the damage and the more specialized the tissue, the greater the immune response is likely to be. With continuous or chronic tissue damage, an autoimmune disease sets in. The Parkinson's neurological manifestations observed in boxer like Ali may well be the result of the immune response to chronic brain trauma (blows to the head).

The damaged tissue protein, acting as an antigen, will prime the tissue macrophages as they mature as lymphocytes or plasma cells to produce tissue protein-specific antibodies. The T cells will react to the antigen-antibody complexes at the injured tissue site.

Jerne predicted that there is some negative feedback mechanism participating in the immune response, when he postulated the network theory of immune regulation. Taking this into consideration, Lewis et al. stated that if Jerne's prediction is a correct fact, "then the immune stimulation should be undertaken with great caution in the clinical setting, unless concurrent measures of antitumor immune response can be undertaken in the patient during therapy." He emphasized the importance of "regulation of the normal immunity rather than to persistently hyperstimulate in a blind fashion."

Cancer pathogenesis

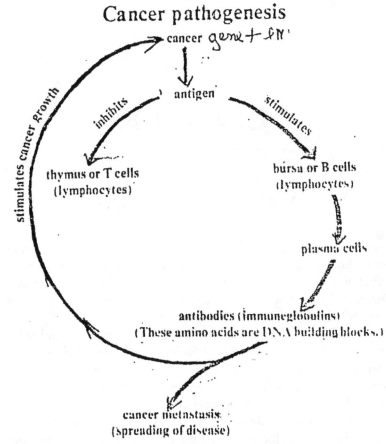

Diagram explaining the interplay of the individual genetic component, with the environment, can promote the development of cancer. Once cancer is generated, it produces antigenic substances that inhibit the T cells, and the cancer cells are not attacked. On the other hand, the same antigen stimulates the B cells to produce antibodies that will not harm the cancer but serve as its nutrient. Excess of antibodies are engulfed by the macrophage, which in turn becomes sensitized with the cancer antigen, and eventually, after reaching their fiftieth division, will transform in situ into metastases. And thus, the vicious cycle continues.

Chapter X

Cancer and Fungus

I have been interested in the cause of diseases for over fifty years, and the field of Pathology has given me that opportunity in the study of cancer. If I could find an answer to the cause of cancer and be able to help to get rid of this dreadful disease, that affects millions of people every year, that would be a dream fulfilled.

Originally, I started by examining living cancer cells suspended in saline solution under the light microscope. Much to my surprise, I observed that the cytoplasm of the cancer cells started to show minute green granules (GG) after 3 minutes of observation. These GG gradually increased in size and appeared to float in the cytoplasm of the cancer cell. The intensity of the green color increased to a brilliant, luminous emerald green color, like fluorescent. As the number of the granules increased, the cell cytoplasm distended and ruptured, releasing the GG into the saline solution. I repeated the experiment with different types of fresh cancer tissues as they came to me from the operating room. The cancer tissues examined were from: cancer of the breast, stomach, colon, lung, ovary, cervix of the uterus, prostate, squamous cell carcinoma of the lip, and one case of leiomyosarcoma of the leg. All showed the same GG when examined as described.

Controls of the same cancer cells from the cancers tissues not exposed to the light did not show the GG. The GG appeared only after exposure to the light. Controls of normal cells suspended in saline and exposed to the light did not show GG.

Subsequently, cancer tissues were fixed in formalin, cut into thin slices, placed on glass slides, stained with Hematoxylin and Eosin, (H&E) and examined under the light microscope. I could not find the GG in the stained tissue slides. Repeated studies of the stained-cancer tissue did not show any GG.

I thought that the GG might have been washed away and lost during the processing of the tissue or that for some reason, the GG were not being stained by the tissue stain being used. I tried again with other stain available, but again the tissue did not show any GG.

What was the nature of these GG? I suspected that the GG were some sort of chlorophyll produced by the primitive cancer cells returning back to a plant physiology when exposed to the light. Little did I know then, how much different my interpretation would be many years later.

Review of the literature on the cause of cancer goes back to the year 1890 when Dr. William Russell, a Pathologist at the School of Medicine in Edinburg presented a paper at the Pathological Society of London where he described his histological findings as "a characteristic organism of cancer".

Dr. Russell observed microscopically, that the infecting organism could be found inside the tissue cells (intracellular) and outside the cells (extracellular). These organisms were round and about half the size of a red blood cell (RBC). He concluded that these bodies suggested a fungal or yeast-like parasite, possible "blastomycete" (a type of fungus). He called these bodies "fuchsine bodies" because of of their bluish-red staining.

Years later, in 1920 an Obstetrician, Dr. James Young, from Scotland grew a pleomophic bacteria from various cancers. The microbe manifested as coccoid (round forms) and yeast-like forms. He called the microbe "spore forms" and "spores balls".

IN 1932, Dr. Royal Reymond Rife, a research Pathologist, isolated a organism from tissue from human breast cancer. He injected this organism into 412 rats, and all the rats developed cancer. Finally,he isolated the organism from the tumors which grew on the rats, and injected the isolated organism into new healthy rats, all the rats developed cancer, and so, he fulfilled Koch's postulate. Rife named the organism, Cryptocides Primordiales.

Late in the 1940's, Dr. Virginia Livingston discovered the cancer microbe. With the help of Alexander Jackson, a microbiologist, they confirmed the microbe to be filterable. Further information on Livingston books on the cancer microbe: Cancer: A New Breakthrough (1972, and The Conquest of Cancer (1984).

At about that time, in 1983, Dr. Tullio Simoncini, an Italian doctor, specialized in Oncology, presented his idea that "cancer and tumors are the result of fungal infections. He demonstrated how he treated and cured cancer patients with solutions of sodium bicarbonate via a catheter. He noted that the tumors disappeared within weeks. (sodium bicarbonate is a strong antifungal). In his published book, "Cancer is a Fungus-The revolution in the Therapy of

Tumors", Dr. Simoncini presents cases of cancer responding by being cured with his sodium bicarbonate treatments.

Unfortunately for Dr. simoncini, The Italian Medical Society opposed his ideas and treatment as illegal and dangerous, by not following the accepted method of cancer treatment. The situation was resolved by taking away the medical license of Dr. Simoncini.

Currently, Dr. Simoncini continues to promote his work via the internet, and by giving lectures about his treatments, and by instructing people with cancer how they can help themselves.

There are other reports of medical doctors supporting the idea that fungus might be the cause of cancer.

In 1983 I presented a paper on my work on, "The Effect of Ozone/Oxygen (O3/O2) Gas Mixture directly Injected Into the Mammary Carcinoma of the C3H/HEJ Mouse", at the Sixth Ozone World Congress, held in Washington, D.C., on May 23-26, 1983. My findings are reported in this book.

In 1085, the above mentioned paper was published in the Journal of Holistic Medicine, Vol. 7 NO 1 Spring/Summer 1985.

I continued my work on cancer with detailed histological examination of multiple slides of H&E stained cancer tissues of various organs as mentioned before, (cancer of the breast, lung, stomach, colon, ovary, prostate, squamous carcinoma of the lip, and a leiomyosarcoma).

By examining under high magnification(oil immersion) of the light microscope numerous stained slides of the cancers previously noted, I found most of the cancer cells and macrophages to have a great number of round, cocci, organism within their cytoplasm. These bacteria-like organisms were not particularly stained by the regulat H&E tissue stain, but were noted by being outlined by the stained surrounded tissue. These bacteria-like forms could be easily missed, if higher magnification withoil immersion was not used.

Years later, re-examination of the photographs of human cancer tissue microscopic findings and comparing them with the pictures of the living cancer cell in mice, represented by what I called at that time Green Granules (GG) are in my opinion most likely to be, one and the same kind of organism. The fact that these organisms did not stain by the usual laboratory stain for tissues, I interpret it to be, due probably to a thicker wall of the infectious organism, not readily absorbing the used stain pigment. I interpret these organisms as most likely to be spores, as in fungus spores. It is important to further investigate this possibility by doing cancer tissue cultures looking for fungus.

Other studies of the mice mammary carcinoma by electron microscopy demonstrated not only cancer cell membrane showing viral budding, but also I found a single free budding organism, as seen in fungus, like Candida in certain conditions. (see electron Photograph).

Also, I found by electron microscopy in a case of human ovarian carcinoma after the tissue was exposed to light prior to processing, an interesting honey-comb-like structure resembling quantosomes. If this structure is not an artifact, could it be that the light exposure provoked the cancer cell to complete the plant physiology by producing a quantosome since already cancer cells have a plant physiology? I believe it is possible, but further studies are necessary. It could be an interesting project.

Based on my findings of: examination of living cancer cells, both in mice and in human cancers, under light microscopy, and by electron microscopy studies, it is my conclusion that fungus may cause cancer. But the absolute answer is by culturing cancer tissue and finding fungus that when injected into healthy rats or mice produces cancer, replicating Dr. Royal Reymond Rife experiments.

Unusual Skin Fungus Infection and Clinical Manifestations.

I will briefly describe an often unrecognized skin infection by Candida Albicans. It may affect predominantly female over 40 years of age, who had a previous yeast infection, such as vagina yeast infection. The patient may appear healthy but, her immune system is already compromised.

They will visit the doctor's office complaining of tiredness, lack of energy, and not being able to sleep well. Some may complain of losing their hair and of having itchy skin rashes or hives in their upper back, arms or legs. Sometimes they complain of temporary painful joints. These patients have good appetite, preferring to eat sweets, carbohydrates, and are always tired.

Upon physical examination the skin lesions hives-like depending on the age of the lesion, may appear reddish reddish when recent, later on become liht brown. Some may show scratches marks, or some sticky exudates when fresh, or a bloody crust. When palpated the lesions are firm and nodular measuring about five mm in size.

Microscopic examination of scrapings from the lesion suspended in saline solution may rarely show yeasts. These patients usually have a generalize fungus infection represented by the clinical symptoms and physical findings. These findings are the result of the fungus infection and fungemia (fungus infection of the blood) in the form of metastatic itchy skin lesions and mycotoxins. This condition, if not treated properly, the patient can become progressively incapacitated, to the point of not being able to carry on the normal daily activities. The patient can be treated with strong antifungal that are absorbed into the blood stream in order to have an effective result. These patients are not to be treated with antibiotics or cortisone, doing so will aggravate the condition.

If a biopsy of the lesion is to be done, it is recommended that the laboratory be contacted in advance, since not all laboratories are equipped to do tissue culture for fungus and tissue stain for fungus. The tissue specimen must br properly marked "for fungus culture and tissue stain for fungus".

Without delay, even before the diagnosis is confirmed by the laboratory tests, that sometimes may come as negative for fungus, it is essential that the patient be placed on an antifungal diet, since fungus lives on starches and sugar. It is essential to follow the diet strictly, even with antifungal medication, if the diet is not followed, the treatment will not be effective.

This is the antifungal diet: The patient is allowed to eat the following: fish, poultry and preferable grass-fed beef (to avoid the mycotoxins, toxins produced by the fungus that usually contaminates the grain they are fed), eggs, vegetables such as avocados. Broccoli, cabbage, water crest, carrots, egg plant, lettuce, tomato, collar greens, onion, garlic, zucchini, sweet potato, summer and winter squash, alfalfa sprouts, spinash, celery, kale, kelp, and in general all green vegetables. Also fresh nuts as: almonds, pecan, walnuts, almond butter. Drink pure water, fresh carrot juice with added celery, beet, onion and a clove of garlic. Drink green tea, water with added one teaspoon full of unfiltered apple cider vinegar. Use cold pressed olive oil, Use flax seed oil, omega 3.

Fruits allowed: grapefruit, lime, lemons, green apples, all kind of berries: strawberries, blue berries, etc.

Not allowed: any kind of sugars including the artificial sweeteners, sweets of any kind, chocolate, ice cream, cake or pastries, alcoholic drinks, soft drinks, fruit juices, coffee, rice, wheat, bread of any kind, no grains, cereals, potato, pasta, spaghetti, peanut or peanut butter (danger of myco-toxins present) mushrooms, fruits. Do not use vegetables oils or trans-fats.

If the patient follows the anti fungus diet strictly as described above, there should be a dramatic improvement of the symptoms with returning of well feeling within two weeks of starting the diet. This is proof that the condition is caused by a fungus: Candida. Now is the time to continue with the diet, because the battle with the fungus is not over. If the patient starts eating the food not allowed, the symptoms will return with double intensity. Strict compliance to the diet is necessary to continue to feel well.

The patient needs to see his/her physician for antifungus prescription therapy if that is the way they want to go, since strong antifungus medication that is absorbed into the blood stream are only obtained by a doctor's prescription.

The patient has the option, after discussing his condition with the doctor to continue with the natural way of treatment, by using the antifungus diet as described above and by using antifungus medications easily obtainable at health food stores. This disease, if not treated properly can progressively incapacitate the patient to the point of not being able to carry the normal daily activities. Even after the proper treatment with antifungus, the patent must continue with the antifungus diet, otherwise the symptoms will recur. The antifungus diet is essential, and to be continued, whether whether the patient is being treated with antifungal or not.

Via the internet, the patient can much information about how to go the natural oral remedies way. Some of the products that kill fungus are: Oil of oregano, olive leaf extracts, caprilic acid, Pau d'arco, garlic eaten fresh. The oral antifungus should not be taken for over a two weeks period at a time. Discontinue for a while, and alternate with a different antifungal, so the fungus do not become resistant to it. The patient is to continue with the antifungus diet all the time. The patient is to check with his doctor for advise and management of his condition and let the physician know if any, what medication he is taking.

Together with the diet, it is necessary for the patient to help his body with the elimination of toxins, (mycotoxins produced by the fungus). This can be accomplished by using Psyllium Husks mixed in water before bedtime, (PM). It will help to eliminate toxins and regulate bowel movements. Read the instructions and follow it, before taking the Psyllium. Make sure to take plenty of water. Psyllium swells, it is a bulking agent. It helps in the cleaning process.

Also it is necessary for the patient to restore the intestinal flora, that will be altered by the antifungus medication. It is advisable to take daily in the morning about 15 minutes before breakfast, (AM). Take one or two capsule of bacillus acidophylus to restore the intestinal flora. Take the acidophilus at least six hours apart from the psyllium, otherwise it will be eliminated with the psyllium.

During the day, drink 6-8 onces of pure water, it will help to eliminate toxins. Dry brush your skin daily, before taking a shower, it will help to get rid of dead skin cells and open the pores to eliminate toxins. Body massage, by stimulating the lymphatic system also helps in the elimination of toxins. Deep breathing exercises (diaphragmatic breathing) massages your abdominal organs and clear your lungs of stale air.

Avoid food additives, and processed foods. Take supplements as needed: Vitamines A, B complex, C, E, Calcium/Magnesium, Expose your body to the sun for 10 minutes daily to get your vitamin D3, if not possible take the D3 orally, Zinc, Chromium, Selenium, Fish Oil/Omega 3, eat fresh garlic, green tea helps the immune system. Other supplements as needed such as: CoQ10, Alpha Lipoic Acid, Acetyl L—Carnitine, L-Carnitine, Phosphatidyl-Serine, etc

It is necessary to do daily exercises: stretching, core physical exercises and others as walking, riding the bicycle and others such as Tai Chi and Qi-Gong. It is very important not only to take care of your body, but of your mind and spirit, otherwise there will be an imbalance in the whole self, and seed for diseases are created in the form of mental blockages inhibiting the normal functioning. Our bodies can not function properly if we hold hate, if we do not forgive, after all no one is perfect. So Forgive, Do not hate, Do not criticize. It is very important to clear your mind from stress and negative emotions by doing daily 15-30 minutes meditation, it will not only clear your mind of clutter, but relax your body as well.

Keeping yourself in order, keep your house in order, your life and business will be in order. As the saying goes, "As a man thinks, so he is". Proverbs 23:7

Think yourself healthty and successful, and you will be.

Keep your mind free of clutter and of negative thoughts. Smile, look at yourself in the mirror and see a new person: You healthy, full of hidden talents to be unveiled. Go for it!

CONCLUSIONS

Based on my cancer research, clinical observations, and in the cancer literature, I have arrived at the following conclusions about cancer:

1. Cancer is the result of the interplay of the genetic component of the individual and of the environment.
2. Cancer develops as the result of an infection of the cell mitochondria by a compatible infectious agent: virus, bacteria or fungus. This result in a cancer embryo. This occurs in a cancer predisposed individual with a weakened immune system. .
3. Once the above takes place, the cancer behaves as an embryo. It produces fetal antigen that inhibits the the T cells from recognizing cancer as an invader, and thus the cancer is not rejected.
4. Cancer produces wastes, carcinoembryonic antigen, and others that act as antigenic substances. These substances stimulate the B lymphocytes to produce plasma cells. In turn, the plasma cells will produce immuneglobulins or antibodies against the cancer wastes.
5. However, the immunoglobulins will not be detrimental to the cancer tissue; on the contrary, it will serve as nourishment for the cancer, and it will promote cancer growth since cancer thrives on antibodies.
6. A vicious circle starts. Cancer behaves as an autoimmune disease.
7. Cancer thrives not only on antibodies, but on the patient's antibody-coated red blood cells as well.
8. Metastases occur predominantly by in situ transformation of the cancer antigen-prime-aged macrophages (fiftieth division).
9. Once tissue cells reach their fiftieth division (end of a normal cell's life span), the individual is more prone to diseases he/she is genetically predisposed to, and the aging process accelerates since regeneration of healthy tissue is impaired.

10. Cancer cells in saline solution, when exposed to the light, produce green granules (GG) in their cytoplasm. The GG are surrounded by a yellow halo around each resembling fluorescence.

11. Though not yet proven, GG could be a primitive form of chlorophyll produced by a cancer cell when exposed to light, and it is trying to survive in the available environment.

12. Cancer cells suspended in saline solution when examined under the light microscope develop large, brilliant, green granules that increase in size and in numbers until the cell bursts freeing the green granules. These green granules are interpreted as highly suspicious of fugus spores, but since cancer tissue culture was not done for fungus, a conclusive, final diagnostic can not be made.

13. By electron photograph, a quantosome-like particle was found in a human papillary adenocarcinoma after light exposure. The nature or significance is not yet determined.

14. Electron microscopic examination of red blood cells of human female with breast cancer, revealed dense coating of the red blood cells with immunecomplexes. These complexes inhibits the normal exchange of nutrients and the elimination of cell wastes.

15. Electron microscopic examination of red blood cells of the mammary carcinoma of the C3H/HEJ mice, after treatment with Ozone/Oxygen gas mixture injections, revealed clearing of most of the immunecomplexes coating the red blood cell surface.

16. Most cancers and degenerative diseases can be prevented with proper diet and healthy life-style.

17. Mandatory vaccination should be eliminated. In my opinion vaccines, produce the seed for chronic degenerative diseases to develop later on in life. Vaccines in general should be eliminated.

18. Cancer and many chronic degenerative diseases are in our power to prevent or greatly reduce the incidence, by proper living and eating habits. Man created treatments such called preventive vaccination, radiation and chemotherapy are barbaric and should be avoided. Given the proper natural care and nutrition the body is built to heal itself.

It is up to us to be responsible and learn as much as possible, on how to eat healthy and live properly to avoid diseases. We should not depend solely in doctors to tell us how to eat or live, because doctors are not trained to prevent, but to treat the symptoms of already established diseases. Since they do not know the cause of diseases, they do try to treat the symptoms.

Try eating plenty of fresh vegetable eaten raw, not overcooked. Drink fresh vegetable juices. Fresh nuts, fish, as salmon, cod, poultry, whole eggs and grass fed beef. Drink pure water, avoid soft drinks and alcoholic beverages as much as possible. Avoid manufactured ready to eat food, they are saturated with artificial preservatives and sweeteners. Avoid sugars, starches and grains. Sleep 8 hours daily. Exercise daily. Meditate and clear your mind. Try to be kind to your fellow men. Do not hate, it will destroy you. Forgive. Think positive.

There you have it, all in a nut shell. Have a healthy, joyful and productive long life.

It is my hope, that reading this book, have opened your eyes to understanding as how diseases are created, and how you can have a strong impact in preventing most diseases. People are as computer: if you put garbage in, you will get garbage out.

This book is not only intended for medical doctors of all specialties, but also it will be helpful to researchers, biologists, nurses and to the general public interested in learning and desiring to take an active part in their health.

Note. The following is reported as a warning not to do experiments on yourselves or any other person. It could kill you, or damage you for the rest of your life.

This Experiment Almost Killed Me.

My husband mother and her two sisters died of breast cancer. Since we had a daughter, I thought that my husband probably had the gene for cancer in his genome, and if I could develop a vaccine against that gene, later on, if there was need, my serum could protect our daughter agaist breast cancer. I prepared a vaccine from my husband sperm cells. This happened in the early seventies when genetic research was unheard of. I inoculated the vaccine in my left deltoid ares. Within an hour of the inoculation the deltoid area and progressively my left arm became painful, red and swollen.

My collegues joked, "Careful, you may develop an embryoma in your arm." For me it was not a funny matter. Within a week, I started to have incontrollable shivers and felt very cold, not even several blankets helped me to feel comfortable. I felt freezing cold. Symptoms became progressively worst when while resting in bed trying to sleep, my body suddenly bolted into a sitting position with a feeling of terror and of imminent death. I felt in my belly as if life was being cut out of me. My heart galloped wildly. I felt ripples all over within my body, as if my genetic matter was reorganizing from the vaccine stimulus. I was unable to sleep. A few days later, I started to bleed, not only vaginally, but also through my nose and mouth. My body was trying to get rid of the antibodies to the vaccine anyway it could. I was very ill for several weeks, but it took me almost a year to recover. The laboratory tests showed: hemolytic anemia, and a high antinuclear antibody titer. My blood smear showed fragmentation and deformation of my red blood cell and increased number of lymphocytes

Months later I found out that I was not able to have sex, because every time we tried, it was like a buster vaccine. Then all the symptoms recurred as before, but with less intensity. Even with care it was not possible. It made a nightmare of my life and of my husband. I had been very foolish and hasty in my decision. It almost cost me, my life. Still to this day many years later, I am suffering the consequences of the vaccine. I was treated with various medications and also with intravenous injections of a mixture of Ozone/oxygen gases to neutralize the antibodies, but I know, I was saved by the grace of God.

CANCER REFERENCES

Chapter 1

1. p. 3, 73. Taylor, J. H. Asynchronous Duplication of Chromosomes in Cultured Cells of Chinese Hamsters. J. Biophs. Biochemistry. Cytol. 1960; 7: 455-463.
1a. p. 3. Gold, Michael. The Cells That Would Not Die. Science. 1981; 2:28-35.
2. p. 4. Milo, George, E. and Noyes, Inge. Transformation of Human Cells. The Ohio State University Comprehensive Cancer Center. Olacc. Oncology Conference. April 27-28, 1984.
3. p. 43, 49. Hayflick, L. The Cell Biology of Human Aging. N. England J. Med. 1976; 295:1302.
4. p. 4, 49. Hayflick, L. The Limited in Vitro Lifetime of Human Diploid Cell Strains. Exp. Cell Res. 1965; 37:614.
5. p. 4, 49. Hayflick, L., and Moorhead, P. S. The Serial Cultivation of Human Diploid Cell Strains. Exp. Cell Res. 1961; 25:585.
6. p. 5, 44. Birbeck, M. S. C., and Dukes, C. E. Electron Microscopy of Rectal Neoplasms. (Chester Beaty Resh. Inst., London). Proc. Roy. Soc. Med. 1963; 56:793-797.
7. p. 6. Rowley, J. D. Nature. 1973; 243:290.
8. p. 6. Collins, Steven, J., Kuboniski, Ichiro., Miyoski, Isao., Groudine, Mark T. Altered Transcription of the c-abl Oncogene in K-562 and Other Chronic Myelogenous Leukemic Cells. Science. 1984; 225:7274.
9. p. 6, 79. Hamerton, John, L. Chromosomes in Medicine. Little Club Clinic. in Developmental Medicine. No. 5. p. 162. Published by the Medical Advisory Committee of the National Spastic Society in Association with Wm. Heinemann. (Medical Books), Ltd. Printed by the Levenham, Suffolk, England.
10. p. 6. Srinivasan, P. R., and Borek, Ernest. (NY) 1964. Enzymatic Alteration of Nucleic Acid Structure. Science. 1964; 145:548-553.
11. p. 6. Clark, R. L. and Cumley, R. W. 1964-65. Year Book of Cancer. p. 458.

12.   p. 6. Joseph M. Kiely (Mayo Clinic). Hypernephroma. M. Clin. North America. 1966; 50:1067-1083.

12a.   p. 6. Lamb, David. (Inst. od Disesses of the Chest, London). Correlation of Chromosome Counts with Histologic Appearances and Prognosis in Transitional Cell Carcinoma of Bladder. Brit. M. J. 1967; 1:273-277.

12b.   p. 6. Ullmann, Alexander, S., and Ross, Oscar, A. Hyperplasia, Atypism and Carcinoma in Situ in Prostatic Periurethral Glands. (Metropolitan Hospital, Detroit, Michigan) Am. J. Clin. Path. 1967; 47:497-504.

13.   p. 6, 50. Ghadially, F. N. and Parry, E. W. (University of Sheffield) Ultrastructure of Human Hepatocellular Carcinoma and Surrounding Non-Neoplastic Liver. Cancer. 1966; 19:1989-2004.

14.   p. 8. Israel, Lucien, MD. Conquering Cancer. Random House, NY 1970. p. 15, 16, 23, 32.

15.   p. 8, 17, 24, 25. Novikoff and Holtzman. Cells and Organelles. p. 104. Publ. Holt, Rheinhart and Winston, Inc. NY. 1970.

16.   p. 11. Price, V. E., Greenfield, R. E., Sterling, W. R., and MacCardie, R. C. Studies on the Anemia of Tumor-Bearing Animals. III. Localization of Erythrocyte Iron Within the Tumor. J. National Cancer Institute. 1959; 22:877-885.

17.   p. 21. Price, V. E., and Greenfield, R. E. Anemia in Cancer. Advances in Cancer Research. 1958; 5:199-290.

18.   p. 21. Greenfield, R. E., Godfrey, J. E., and Price, V. E. Studies on the Anemia of Tumor-Bearing Animals. I. Distribution of Radiation Following the Injection of Labeled Erythrocytes. J. National Cancer Institute 1958; 21:641-656.

19.   p. 21. Greenfield, R. E., Sterling, W. R., and Price, V. E. Studies on the Anemia of Tumor-Bearing Animals. IV. Distribution of Radio Iron after Extravascular Injection of Labeled Erythrocytes. J. National Cancer Institute. 1960; 24:87-96.

20.   p. 10. Greenfield, R. E., Sterling, W. R., and Price, V. E. Studies on the Anemia of Tumor-Bearing Animals. II. The Mechanisms of Erythrocytes Destruction. J. National Cancer Institute. 1958; 21:1099-1107.

21.   p. 20. Bapson, A. L. and Winnick, F. 1954. Cancer Res. 1954; 14:606.

22.   p. 21. Bush, H. and Green, H. S. N. Studies of the Metabolism of Plasma Proteins in Tumor-Bearing Rats. Yale J. Biol. and Med. 1955; 27:339-349.

23.   p. 21. Campbell, P. N. Protein Synthesis with Special Reference to Growth Processes Both Normal and Abnormal. Advances in Cancer Research. 1958; 5:97-155.

24.   p. 21. Bush, H., Sembonis, S., Anderson, D. C., and Green, H. S. N. Studies on the Metabolism of Plasma Proteins in Tumor-Bearing Rats. II. Labeling of Intracellular Particulates of Tissues by Radioactive Albumin and Globulins. Yale J. Biol. and Med. 1956; 29:105-116.

25.   p. 21. Kent, H. N. and Gey, G. O. 1957. Changes in Serum Proteins During Growth of Malignant Cells in Vitro. Proc. Soc. Exptl. Biol. Med. 1957; 94:205-209.

———

26. p. 21. Greenlees, J., Le Page, G. A. 1955. Protein Turnover on a Study of Host-Tumor Relationships. Cancer Research. 1955; 15:256-262.

27. p. 21. Midler, Tesliak and Morton. 1948. Acta Un. Int. Cancer. 1948; 6:409.

28. p. 23, 48, 63. Winich, Myron. Nutrition and Cancer. A Wiley Interscience Publication. 1977.

29. p.23,24.Korngold,L.and Pressman,D.1954.Localization of Antilymphosarcoma Antibodies in the Murphy Lymphosarcoma of the Rat. Cancer Research. 1954; 14:96-102.

30. p.24.Morton, H., Pasieka, A. E., and Morgan, J. F. 1956. The Nutrition of Animal Tissues Cultured in Vitro. III. Use of a Depletion Technique for Determining Specific Nutritional Requisites. J. Biophyp. Cytol. 1956; 2:589-596.

31. p. 10, 11, 12, 13. Pendersen, P. L. 1978. Tumor Mitochondria and the Bionergetics of Cancer Cells. Progress in Experimental Tumor Research. Editor: F. Homburger, Cambridge, Massachusetts. Publ: S. Karger, Basel, Switzerland. 1978; 22:190-276. p. 194, 195, 211, 216, 227, 228, 251.

32. p. 10. Science. 1980; 210:1334.

34. p. 11. Irwin, C. C. and Malkin, L. L. Differences in the Total Mitochondrial Proteins and Mitochondrially Synthesized Proteins and Mitochondrially Synthesized Proteins from Rat Liver and Harris Hepatoma. Fed. Proc. Fed. Am. Socs. Exp. Biol. 1976; 35:1583.

35. p. 12. Mills, Dan, C. (Washington University) 1963. Endometrial Cancer in Patients Previously Irradiated for Cervical Cancer. Obstetrics and Gynecology. 1963; 22:280-283.

36. p. 12. Trump, Benjamin, F., and Jones, Raymond T. 1978. Diagnostic Electron Microscopy. John Wiley & Sons, Inc. Vol. I. 1978. p. 14-17.

37. p. 13. Borst, P. and Kroom, A. M. Mitochondrial DNA: Physicochemical Properties, Replication Genetic Function. University of Amsterdam, the Netherlands. p. 155.

38. p. 13. Mitochondria Inheritance. Biology of Microorganism. Brocks, Thomas, D. Second Edition Prentice-Hall Inc. Englehood, NJ. 1974. p. 439.

39. p. 13, 14. Lehninger, Albert, L. Biochemistry. Worth Publishers, Inc. Second Edition. 1975. p. 939, 940.

40. p. 14. Lau, B. W. C. and Chan, S. H. P. 1984. Efflux of Adenine Nucleotides in Mitochondria from Rat Tumor Cells of Varying Growth Rates. Cancer Research. 1984; 44:4458-4464.

41. p. 14. Somlo and Fukuhara. 1965. Biosynthesis of Mitochondrial Cytochromes in Sacharomyces.

42. p. 14. Lukins et al., 1966. Swift et al. 1968.

43. p.15. Reilly and Sherman, 1965.

44. p.15. Polakis and Bartley, 1965; Jaraman et al., 1966.

45. p.16. Tzagoloff, Alexander. Mitochondria. Ed. Phillip Siekevitz. Rockefeller University, NY. Plenum Press. NY. London. Sec. Print. 1983. p. 131.

46. p. 17. Tandler, Bernard and Happel, Charles, L. Mitochondria. Academic Press. NY. p. 33.

47. p. 24. Cancer Research. October 1984; 44:4461.

48. p. 24, 27, 33. Robins, S. I., Contran, RS. Pathologic Basis of Disease. Carcinoembryonic Antigen. Second Edition. W. B. Saunders Co. 1979. p. 81.

49. p. 24, 33. Thompson, D. M. P., Krupey, J., Freedman, S. D., and Gold, P. 1969. The Radioimmunoassay of Circulating Carcinoembryonic Antigen of the Human Digestive System. Proc. Nat. Acad. Sci. USA. 1969; 64:161-167.

50. p. 24, 33. Hansen, H. J., Snyder, J. J., Miller, E., et al. Carcinoembryonic Antigen (CEA) Assay-A Laboratory Adjunct in the Diagnosis and Management of Cancer. Human Pathology. 1974; 5:139-147.

51. p. 25. Gold, P. and Freedman, S. D. 1965. Demonstration of Tumor-Specific Antigens in Human Colonic Carcinomata by Immunological Tolerance and Absorption Techniques. J. Exptl. Med. 1965; 122:467-481.

52. p. 25. Gold, P. and Freedman, S. O. 1965. Specific Carcinoembryonic Antigens of the Human Digestive System. J. Exptl. Med. 1965; 122:467-481.

53. p. 25. Slater, H. S. and Coligan, G. E. 1975. Electron Microscopy and Physical Characterization of the Carcinoembryonic Antigen. Biochemistry. 1975; 14:2323-2330.

54. p. 25. Egan, Marianne L., Coliga, John E., Pritchard, David G., Schnute, William Jr. C., Todd, Charles W. 1976. Cancer Research. 1976; 36:3482-3485.

55. p. 25. Technical Methods and Procedures. American Association of Blood Banks. Chicago, Illinois. 1973.

56. p. 25. Encyclopedia of Immunohematology. Pfizer Diagnostic Division. 1973.

57. p. 25. Blood Group Antigens and Antibodies as Applied to Blood Transfusion. Ortho Diagnostic Division. Raritan, NY. 1960.

58. p. 25. Davidsohn, I. 1972. Early Immunologic Diagnosis and Prognosis of Carcinoma. Am. J. Clin. Pathol. 1972; 57:715.

59. p. 25. Gold, J. M., Freedman, S. O., Gold, P. 1972. Human Anti CEA Antibodies Detected by Radioimmunoelectrophoresis. Nature. 1972; 60:234.

60. p. 26. Cellular Antigens and Disease. American Association of Blood Banks. Ed. E. A. Sterns, PhD, 1977, p. 6-12.

61. p. 27, 31. Noto, T. A., Miale, J. B. and Riekers, H. 1964. Quantitation of Human Chorionic Gonadotropin in Urine Using the Slide Immunological Test for Pregnancy. Am. J. Obstetrics and Gynecology. 1964; 90:859.

62. p. 27. Aging and its Chemistry. Proceeding of the Third Arnold O. Beckman Conference in Clinical Chemistry. Albert A. Dietz, Editor. The American Association for Clinical Chemistry. Washington DC. 1725 K St. NW Washington DC, 2006. p. 36. 1979.

63. p. 27. Lesher, S., Grahn, D., and Sallese, A. 1957. Amyloidosis in Mice Exposed to Daily Gamma Irradiation. J. National Cancer Institute. 1957; 19:119-1131.

64. p. 29. Marx, Jean L. 1982. Monoclonal Antibodies in Cancer. Science. 1982; 216:283-285.

65. p. 29. Preuss, Paul. 1983. The Shape of Things to Come. Science. 1983. Dec. AAAS. p. 80-87.

66. p. 30. Strelkankas, Anthony J., Wilson, Barry S., Dray, Sheldon. 1975. Nature, 1975; 258:331-332.

67. p. 30. Lewis, J., Whang, J.,m Nagel, B. J., Oppenheim, J. J. and Perry, S. 1966. Am. J. Obstetrics and Gynecology. 1966; 96:287-290.

68. p. 30. Han, T. 1975. Immunology. 1975; 29:509-515.

69. p. 30. McManus, Linda, Naughton, Michael A., Martinez-Hernandez, Antonio. 1976. Cancer Research. 1976; 36:3476-3481.

70. p. 31. Gold, P. & Freedman, S. O. 1965. Demonstration of Tumor-Specific Antigens in Human Colonic Carcinomata by Immunological Tolerance and Absorption Techniques. J. Exp. Med. 1965; 121:439.

71. p. 31. Gold, P. & Freedman, S. O. 1965. Specific Carcinoembryonic Antigens of the Human Digestive System. J. Exp. Med. 1965; 122:467.

72. p. 31. Bessell, E. M., Thomas, P., and Westwood, J. H. 1975. Multiple Smith-Degradations of Carcinoembryonic Antigen (CEA) and of Asialo CEA. Carbohydr. Res. 1975; 45:257.

73. p. 31. Morris, J. E., Egan, M. L., and Todd, C. W. 1975. The Binding of Carcinoembryonic by Antibody and its Fragments. Cancer Res. 1975; 35:1804.

74. p. 31. L. C. Yeoman and Bush, H. 1978. Oncofetal Chromatin Proteins. Scand. J. Immunology. Vol. 7 Supplement 6. 1978. p. 47-61.

75. p. 31. Shively, J. E. and Todd, C. W. 1978. Carcinoembryonic Antigen. Scan. J. Immunol. Vol. 7, Supplement 6. 1978. p. 19-31.

76. p. 31. Bradbury, J. T. and Gaplerud, C. P. 1963. Serum Chorionic Gonadotropin Studied in Sensitized Rh-Negative Patients. Obstetrics and Gynecology. 1963; 21:330.

77. p. 31. McCarthy, C. and Pennington, G. W. 1964. Maternal Chronic Gonadotropin Concentration as an Aid to the Antenatal Prediction of Hemolytic Disease of the Newborn Infant. Am. J. Obstetrics and Gynecology. 1964; 89:1069.

78. p. 31. Goplerud, C. P. and Bradbury, J. T. 1965. Quantitative Serum Chorionic Gonadotropin. Studies in Abnormal Pregnancy. Am. J. Obstetrics and Gynecology. 1965; 9:23.

79. p. 32. Adcock, E. W., Teasdale, F., August, C. S., Cox, S., Mechia, G., Battaglia, F. C., and Naughton, M. A. 1973. Human Chorionic Gonadotropin its Possible Role in Maternal Lymphocyte Suppression. Science. 1973; 181:845-847.

80. p. 32. Masson, P. L., Delire,M., Cambiaso, C. L. 1977. Nature. 1977; 266:542-543.

81. p. 32. Baldwin, R. N., Price, M. R., Robins, R. A. 1972.Nature New Biol. 1972; 238:185-187.

82.   p. 33. Neville, A. M. 1981. Carcinoembryonic Antigen the Current Status. (editorial). Arch. Pathol. Lab. Med. 1981; 105:285-282.

83.   p. 33, 34. Ruff, M. R., Pert, C. B. 1984. Small Cell Carcinoma of the Lung: Macrophage-Specific Antigens Suggest Hemopoietic Stem Cell Origen. Science. 1984; 225:1034-1036.

84.   p. 33, 34. Currie, G. A. and Alexander, P. 1974. Spontaneous Shedding of TSTA by Viable Sarcoma Cells: Its Possible Role in Facilitating Metastatic Spread. Brit. J. Cancer. 1974; 29:72-75.

85.   p. 33. Rowan, R. A., Masek, M. A., Thompson, J. M., and Frenster, J. H. 1975. Electron Microscopic Localization of Acid Phosphatase Activity Within Hodgkin's Disease Lymph Nodes. Preoc. Am. Ass. Cancer Res. 1975; 16:10-11.

86.   p. 34. Sjogren, H. D., Hellstrom, I., Bansal, S. C., Hellstrom, K. E. 1971. Suggestive Evidence that the Blocking Antibodies of Tumor-Bearing Individuals May be Antigen-Antibody Complexes. Proc. Nat. Acad. Sci. USA. 1971; 68:1372-1375. (NYAS Vol. 277 p. 49)

87.   p. 34. Masek, M. A., Rhoades, D. J., Frenster, J. H. 1973. In Vivo Macrophage Interactions with Lymphocytes in Hodgkin's Disease. Proc. Amer. Ass. Cancer Research. 1973; 14:8-9.

88.   p. 34. Kirchner, H., Glaser, M., and Herberman, R. B. 1975. Suppression of Cell-Mediated Tumor Immunity by Corynebacterium parvum. Nature. (London). 1975; 257:396-398.

89.   p. 34. Catovsky, D. 1975. T Cell Origin of Acid Phosphatase Positive Lymphoblasts. Lancet, 1975; 2:327-328.

90.   p. 34. Kadin, M. E., Newcomb, S. R., Gold, S. B., and Stites, D. P. 1974. Origin of Hodgkin's Cells. Lancet. 1974; 2:167-168.

91.   p. 34. Maylight, G. M. U., Gutterman, J. U., Hersh, E. M. and McBride, C. M. 1973. Antigen Solubilized from Human Solid Tumors: Lymphocyte Stimulation and Delayed Hypersensitivity. Nature. (New Biol.) 1973; 243:188-190.

92.   p. 35. Osborne, D. J. 1984. Concepts of Target Cells in Plant Cell Differentiation. 1984; 14(3):161-169. Elsever Scientific Publishers, Ireland, Limited.

93.   p. 35. Woodruff, M. F. A. 1983. Cellular Heterogeneity in Tumors. Br. J. Cancer. 1983; 47:589-594.

94.   p. 35. Buick, R. N. and Pallack, M. N. 1984. Perceptives on Clonogenic Tumor Cells. 1984; 44 (No. 11); 4909-5462. p. 4916.

95.   p. 46. Gullino, M. Pietro. 1980. Influence of Blood Supply on Thermal Properties and Metabolism of Mammary Carcinomas. (NCI). Annals NYAS. 1980; 335:1-21. p. 21.

96.   p. 43. Oppenheimer, Enid T., Willhite, Margaret Purdy, Stout, Arthur, Denishefky, I., and Fishman, M. Meyer. (Columbia University) 1964. Comparative Study of Effects of Imbedding Cellophane and Polysterene Films in Rats. 1964. Cancer Research. 1964; 24:379-387.

Chapter II

97. p. 3, 4, 5, 49. Heyflick, Leonard, Moohead, P. S. 1961. The Serial Cultivation of Human Diploid Cell Strains, Exp. Cell Res. 1961; 25:585-627.

98. p. 49, 53. Heyflick, Leonard. Aging its Chemistry. Ed. Albert A Dietz. Publ: American Association for Clinical Chemistry Inc. 1980. p. 227.

99. p. 49. Fogh, J. F., and Lund, R. O. 1957. Continuous Cultivation of Epithelial Cell Strain (FL) from Human Ammniotic Membrane. Proc. Soc. Exp. Biol. & Med. 1957; 94:532.

100. p. 49. Gey, G. O. 1955. Some Aspects of the Constitution and Behavior of Normal and Malignant Cells Maintained in Continuous Culture. Harvey Lectures. 1954-55; 50:154.

101. p.49.Gey,G.O.,andGey,M.K.1936.TheMaintenanceofHumanNormalCellsand TumorCellsinContinuousCulture.I.PreliminaryReport:CultivationofMesoblastic Tumors and Normal Tissue. Am. J. Cancer. 1936; 27:45. (from tissue cult. book).

102. p. 51, 75. McCarthy, William, C. 1922. Factors Which Influence Longevity in Cancer. Ann. Surg. 1922; 76:9-12.

103. p. 51. Moore, O. S. and Foote, F. W. 1949. The Relatively Favorable Prognosis of Medullary Carcinoma of the Breast. 1949; 2:635-642.

104. p. 53, 54. Albores-Saavedra, George, Rose, George G., Ibanez, Michael L., Russell, Williams O., Grey, Clifford E., and Dmochowski, Leon. (University of Texas: MD Anderson Hospital and Tumor Institute) 1964. The Amyloid in Solid Carcinoma of the Thyroid Gland: Staining Characteristics, Tissue Culture, and Electron Microscopic Observations. 1964-65 Series Year Book of Cancer. Edit. Clark Cumley. Year Book Publishers. Chicago, Illinois. p. 336-338.

105. p. 54. Zarling, J. M. and Tevethia, S. S. 1973. J. National Cancer Institute. 1973; 50:149-157.

106. p. 54. Kaplan, Alan M., Morahan, Page S. 1976. Macrophage Mediated Tumor Cell Toxicity. International Conference on Immunobiology of Cancer. Annals of the New York Academy of Sciences. 1976; 276:134-145.

107. p. 54. Hellstrom and Hellstrom. Cell Mediated Immunity. 1976. International Conference on Immunobiology of Cancer. Annals NYAS. 1976; 276:316-327.

108. p. 54. Lewis, M. G., Hartman, D., and Jerry, L. M. 1976. Antibodies and Anti-Antibodies in Human Malignancy: An Expression of Deranged Immune Regulation. Annals NYAS. 1976; 276:316-327. p. 326.

109. p. 56. Hakkinen, I. P. T. 1966. Immunochemical Method for Detecting Carcinomatous Secretion from Human Gastric Juice. Scandinav. J. Gastroenterol. 1966; 153:1252-1254.

110. p. 56. McClintock, Barbara. 1951. Chromosoma Organization and Genetic Expression. 1951. Cold Spring Harbor Symposia on Quantitative Biology. 1951; 16:13-47.

111. p. 56. Federoff, Nina V. 1984. Transposable Genetic Elements in Maize. 1984. Scientific American. 1984; 250:84-94.

112. p. 57, 66. Fidler, Isaiah J. Chairman of the Department of Cell Biology of the University of Texas. 1984. Abstract International Symposium on Cancer Research. Washington DC. September 1984. Sponsored by the National Foundation for Cancer Research. Scientific Director: Albert Szent-Gyorgi. Woods Hole, Massachusetts.

113. p. 65. DiBerardino, Marie A., Hoffner, Nancy J. 1983. Gene Reactivation in Erythrocytes; Nuclear Transplantation in Oocytes and Eggs of Rana. Science. 1983; 7:862-864.

114. p. 58. Leibovich, S. J. and Ross. 1975. The Role of Macrophage in Wound Repair: A Study with Hydrocortizone and Antimacrophage Serum. Am. Jour. Pathology. 1975; 78:71-92.

115. p. 58. Ross, R. et al. 1982. Growth Factors and Cell Proliferation. Annals New York Academy of Science. 1982; 397:18-24.

116. p. 58. Kohler, N., and Lipton, A. 1974. Platelets as Source of Fibroblast Growth-Promoting Activity. Expe. Cell. Res. 1974; 87:297-301,

117. p. 58. Ross, R., Glomset, J., Kariya, B., and Harker, L. A. 1974. Platelet-Dependent Serum Factor that Stimulates the Proliferation of Arterial Smooth Muscle Cells in Vitro. Proc. Natl. Acad. Sci. USA. 1974; 71:1207-1210.

118. p. 58. Owen, Albert J., Panagiotes, Pantazis., Antoniades, N. Harry. 1984. Simian Sarcoma Virus Transformed Cell Secrete a Mitogen Identical to Platelet-Derived Growth Factor. Science. 1984; 225:54-56.

119. p. 58. Carpenter et al. 1982. Epidermal Growth Factor. NYAS. 1982; 397:11-17.

120. p.59. Poste, George. 1982. Cell Heterogeneity in Malignant Neoplasm. Annals NYAS. 1982; 397:34-48.

121. p. 59. Fidler, I. J., et al. Phenotype Diversity in Murine Melanoma. J. National Cancer Institute. 67:947-946.

122. p. 60. Reif, Arnold E., Dekker, Marcel, Inc. Immunity and Cancer in Man. An Introduction. Immunology Series. Vol. 3. Mallory Institute. Boston, Massachusetts. 1975.

123. p. 60. Gold, P. 1972. Tumor Specific Antigen in GI Cancer. Hospital Practice. February 1972, p. 79-88.

124. p. 60. Constanza, M. E., Saroj, D., Nathason, L., Dule, A., And Schwartz, R. S. 1974. Carcinoembryonic Antigen: Report of a Screening Study. Cancer. 1974; 33:583-590.

125. p. 61. Hakkinen, J., and Vii, Kari S. 1969. Occurrence of Fetal Sulfoglycoprotein Antigen in the Gastric Juice of Patients with Gastric Disease. Ann. Surg. 1969; 169:277-281.

126. p. 62, 63. Kalis, N. 1958. Immunological Enhancement of Tumor Homographs in Mice: A review. Cancer Res. 1958; 18:992-1003.

127. p. 62. Futrell, J. W. and Myers, G. H. 1973. Regional Lymphadenites and Cancer Immunity. Amm. Surg. 1973; 177:1-7.

128. p. 63. Baldwin, R. W., Hopper, D. G. and Pimm, M. V. 1976. Bacillus-Calmette-Guerin Contact Immunotherapy of Local and Metastatic Deposits of Rats Tumors. International Conference on Immunotherapy of Cancer. Annals NYAS. 1976; 277:124-134.

129. p. 63. Gutterman, Jordan U., Mavligit, Giora M., Blumenshein, George., Burgess, Michael A., McBride, Charles M., and Hersh, Evan M. 1976. Immunotherapy of Human Solid Tumors with Bacillus Calmette-Guerin: Prolongation of Disease-Free Interval and Survival in Malignant Melanoma, Breast and Colorectal Cancer. Annals NYAS. 1976; 277:135-159.

130. p. 63. Motomichi Torusori, Mitsuyuki Fukawa, Masaga Nishimura, Hiroaki Harasaki, Shiochi Kai and Jiro Tanaka. 1976. Immunotherapy of Cancer Patients with Bacillus Calmette-Guerin: Summary of Four Years of Experience in Japan. Annals NYAS. 1976; 277:160-186.

131. p. 63. Pinsky, Carl M., Hirshaut, Yashar, Vanebo, Harold J., Fortner, Joseph G., Mike, Valerie, Shottenfeld, David, and Oetgen, Herbert F. 1976. Randomized Trials of Bacillus Calmette-Guerin (Percutaneous Administration) as Surgical Adjuvant Immunotherapy for Patients With Stage II Melanoma. Annals NYAS. 1976; 277:187-194.

132. p. 63. Cunningham, Thomas J., Antemann, Richard, Paonessa, Dominick, Sponzo, Robert W., and Steiner, Deborah. 1976. Adjuvant Immuno-and/or Chemotherapy with Neuromidase-Treated Autogenous Tumor Vaccine and Bacillus Calmette-Guerin for Head and Neck Cancers. Annals NYAS. 1976; 277:339-354.

28. p. 64. Winnick, Myron. Nutrition and Cancer. A Wiley Interscience Publication. 1977.

135. p. 65 Steinenn and Fulginiti. Immunological Disorders. Sauders. 1973.

Chapter III

133. p. 76. Tourine, I. L., Tourino, F., Incefy, G. S. and Good, R. A. 1975. Effect of Thymic Factors on the Differentiation of Human Marrow Cells Into T-Lymphocytes in vitro in Normals and Patients with Immunodeficiencies. Annals NYAS. 1975; 249:335-342.

134. p. 76. Serroce, B., Reme, T., Senelar, R., Delor, B., Dubois, J. B., and Thierry, C. 1975. T-Lymphocyte Maturation and Antitumoral Effect of a Thymic Extract Obtained from a Stimulated Model. Annals NYAS. 1975; 249:328-334.

135. p. 77. Steienm and Fulginiti. Immunological Disorders. Saunders. 1973.

136. p. 68, 69. German, James. 1978. DNA Synthesis, Recombination and Viral Genome Integration. Chromosome and Cancer. The New York Blood Center. Publ. John Wiley and Sons Inc., NY. Vol. I. 1978.

137. p. 77. Homma, T., Kansi, P. J., Yang, C. S., Essex, M. 1984. Lymphomas in Macaques: Association with Virus Human T Lymphothrophic Family. Science. 1984; 225:716-718.

138. p. 77. Persson, Hakan, Leder, Phyllip. 1984. Nuclear Localization and DNA Binding Properties of a Protein Expressed by Human c-Myc Oncogene. Science. 1984; 226:527-528.

139. p. 78. Hsio, L. W., Gattoni-Cella, S., and Weinstein, I. B., 1984. Oncogene-Induced Transportation of $C_3H_{10}T1/2$ Cells is enhanced by Tumor Promoters. Science. 1984; 226:552-555.

140. p. 78. Perry, L. Jeanne, and Wetzel, Ronald. 1984. Disulfide Bond Engineers into T4 Lypozyme: Stabilization of the Protein Toward Thermal Inactivation. Science. 1984; 226:555-557.

141. p. 78. Thorton, J. M., 1981. J. Mol. Biol. 1981; 151:261.

142. p. 78. Anfinsen, C. B., and Scheraga, H. A. 1975. Adv. Prot. Chem. 1975; 29:205.

143. p. 78. Twardzik, Daniel R., Tadaro, George I., Marquardt, Hans, Reynolds, Jr., Fred H., and Stephenson, John R. 1982. Science.1982; 216:894-897.

144. p. 82. Schiemke, Robert T. 1980 Gene amplification and Drug Resistance. Sci. Am. 1980;243:60-69.

145. p.83. Dulbecco, R. 1969. Cell Transformation by the Small DNA Containing Viruses. Harvey Lect. 1969; 63:33-49.

146. p. 83. Vogt. M., Dulbecco, R. 1960, Virus-Cell Interaction with a Tumor-Producing Virus. Proc. Nat. Acad. Sci. (US). 1960; 46:365-370.

147. p. 84. Groce, Carlo M., and Klein, George. 1985. Chromosome Translocations and Human Cancer. Scientific American. 1985; 252:54-60.

148. p. 84. Novich, Richard. 1980. Plasmids. Scientific American. 1980; 243:103-127.

149. p. 85, 89. Marx, Jean L. 1984. Perusing the Myc Gene. Science. 1984; 223:675.

150. p. 85. Feig, L. A., Bast, R. C., Knapp, R. C., Cooper, G. M. 1984. Somatic Activation of K-ras Gene in a Human Ovarian Carcinoma. Science. 1984; 223:698-700.

151. p. 85. 1983. Oncogenes and Platelets Dermal Growth Factors. Science. 1983; July 15, p. 248.

152. p. 86. Downward, J., Yarden, Y., Mayer, E., Scrase, G., Tolty, N., Stockwell, P., Ulrich, A., Schlessinger, J. Waterfield, MD. 1984. Nature. 1984; 307:521.

153. p. 86. Marx, Jean L. 1984. Oncogene Linked to Growth Factor Receptor. Science. 1984; 223:806.

154. p. 87. Borek, C. and Hall, E. J. 1982. Annals NYAS. 1982; 397:193-210.

155. p.88. Borek, C., Hall, E. J., and Rossi, H. H. 1978. Malignant Transformation in Cultured Hamster Embryo Cells Produced by X-rays, 450 Kev Monoenergetic Neutrons and Heavy Ions. Cancer. Res. 1978; 38:2997-3005.

156. p. 77, 88. Borek, C., Guernsey, D. L. 1981 Thyroid Hormone Modulated Neoplastic Transformation in Vitro. J. Supramol. Struc. and Cell. Biochem. Suppl. 1981; 5218.

157. p. 88. German, James. 1974. Chromosomes and Cancer. Vol. I. Edit. John Wiley and Son. 1974.

(?)   Weinberg, Robert A. 1983. A Molecular Basis of Cancer. Scientific Am. 1983; 249:126-142.

160. p. 90. Temin, H. M. Nature of the Provirus of Rous Sarcoma. National Cancer Institute Monog. 17:557-570.

161. p. 90. Baltimore, D. 1970. RNA Dependant DNA Polymerase in Virions of RNA Tumor Viruses. Nature. 1970; 226:1209-1211.

162. p. 91. Medawar, P. B. and Medawar, J. S. 1977. The Life Science. Publ. Harpers and Row, NY. 1977. p. 92.

163. p. 93, 96, 173, 210. Watson, James D. 1976. Molecular Biology of the Gene. Third Edition. Publ. W. A. Benjamin, Inc. 1976. p. 614, 211.

Chapter IV

164. p. 96. Milstein, Cesar. 1980. Monoclonal Antibodies. Scientific American. 1980; 243:66-74.

165. p. 97, 98, 173. Lehninger, Albert L. Second Edition. 1975. Worth Publishers Inc. 1975. p. 729, 902, 903, 913, 914, 951.

166. p. 99. Tseng, Howard. 1980. Atlas of Ultrastructure. Publ. Appleton-Century-Crofts, New York. 1980. p. 90.

167. p. 99. Rhodin, W. B. 1963. An Atlas of Ultrastructure. Saunders Company. 1963. p. 90.

168. p. 99, 100, 101. Stephen and North. Biology. 1974. Publ. Wiley and Sons, Inc. p. 130.

169. p. 100. Chlorophyll Organization and Energy Transfer in Photosynthesis. Ciba Foundation Symposium 61. 1979. Exerta Medica. Amsterdam. NY. p. 55, 346, 347, 82, 67, 68, 346, 347, 2.

170. p. 102, 104. Brock, Thomas D. Biology of Microorganism. Publ. Prentice-Hall. 1974. p. 204-205.

171. p. (?) Yamanaka, N. and Deamer, D. 1974. Physiol. Chem. Phys. 1974; 6:95-106.

172. p.107. Dionisi, Ornella, Galeotti, Tomaso, Terranova, Tullio, and Azzi, Angelo. 1975. Biochemica et Biophysica Acta. 1975; 403:292-300.

173. p. 107. Mounolou et al. and Swift et al. 1968. Mitochondrial DNA Physicochemical Properties, Replication and Genetic Function. Publishers. P. Borst and A. M. Kroom, Amsterdam. The Netherlands. 1968.

174. p. 108. Calvin, M. 1959. Evolution of Enzymes and the Photosynthetic Apparatus. Science. 1959; 130:1170.

175. p. 108. Hoppe, Walter, Lohmann, Walfgang., Markl, Hubert., Ziegler, Hubert. 1983. Byophysics. Publ. Springer—Verlag. Berlin. Heidelberg, New York, Tokyo. 1983. p. 515-517.

176. p. 108. Guttman, Burton S. Biological Principles. 1971. Publ. W. A. Benjamin, Inc. NY. p. 77.

177. p. 108. Ford, James M., and Monroe, James E. Living Systems. 1974. Second Edition. Publ. Canfiels Press. San Francisco. A Department of Harper and Row. Publishers, Inc. NY. Evanston, London. 1974. p. 182, 183, 184.

178. p. 108. Milne, Lorus J., and Milne, Margary. Plant Life. Prentice-Hall, Inc. Englewood Cliffs, NJ. 1959. p. 52-53.

179. p. 109. Staehelin, L. A. and Artzen, C. J. 1979. Chlorophyll Organization and Energy Transfer in Photosynthesis. Ciba Foundation Symposium #81, 1979. Exerta Medica. Amsterdam, NY. p. 166.

Chapter V

180. p. 111, 117, 156. Suthers, Roderick A., and Gallant, Roy A. Biology the Behavioral View. 1973. Xerox College Publishing. Lexington, Massachusetts. Toronto. p. 386, 421.

181. p. 112, 113, 114, 115, 116. Eugene H., and Schaeffer, Riley. Chemistry. 1973. Publ. Harper and Row. p. 439, 443, 463, 464, 586-590, 536, 231, 237.

182. p. 116. Shodell, Michael. 1982. The Curative Light. Science.1982; 3(no.3):46-51.

183. p.113.Etkin,William.,Devlin,RobertM.andBouffard,ThomasG.BiologyofHuman Concern. 1972. Publ. J. B. Lippincott Company. Philadelphia, NY. Toronto. p. 225.

184. p. 113. Gullino, Pietro M. 1980. Annals NYAS. 1980; 335:1-21.

185. p. 120. Song, Chang W., Kang, Man S., Rhee, Young S., and Levitt, Seymor H. 1980. Effect of Hyperthermia on Vascular Function in Normal and Neoplastic Tissues. Thermal Characteristics of Tumors: Applications in Detection and Treatment. Annals NYAS. 1980; 335:35-47.

186. p. 121. Wolanski, Bohdan S. 1873. Negative Staining of Plants Agents. Mycoplasma and Mycoplasma-like Agents of Human, Animal and Plant Diseases. Annals NYAS. 1970; 174:675-689.

187. p. 121. Livingston, Afton Munk, Livingston-Wuerthle-Caspe, Virginia, Hackson, Eleanor, and Wolter, Gerhart H. 1970. Toxic Fractions Obtained from Tumor Isolates and Related Clinical Implications. Annals of the New York Academy of Sciences. 1970; 174:675-689.

Chapter VI

196. p. 120. Diet, Nutrition, and Cancer. National Academic Press. 1982. Washington DC. p. 6-11.

197. p. 120. Babson, A. L., and Winnick, T. 1954. Cancer Res. 1954; 14:606.

198. p. 121. White and Andervont. 1943. Casein Diet in C3H mice (?)

199. p. 121. White and White. 1944. Lysine def. Diet. F. R. White and M. Belkin. J. National Cancer Institute. 1945; 5:261.

200. p. 121. Kolonel et al. 1981. Nutrition and Cancer.

201. p. 121. Howell, 1974.

202. p. 121. Dali, 1975. Meat and Ca of Prostate. (?)

203. p. 122.Committe on Cancer. Diet, Nutrition, and Cancer. National Academy of Science Press. Washington DC. 1982. p. 6-11.

204. p. 122. Huggins, C., and Yang, N. C. 1962. Induction and Extinction of Mammary Cancer. Science. 1962; 137:257.

205. p. 122. Tannenbaum, A. 1942. The Genesis and Growth of Tumors. II. Effects of Caloric Restrictions. Cancer Research. 1942; 2:460-467.

206. p. 122. Tannenbaum, A. The Genesis and Growth of Tumors. II. Effects of Caloric Restrictions. Relationship of Body Weight to Cancer Incidence. Arch. Path. 1940; 30:509-517.

207. p. 122. Vischer, P., Ball, M. B., Barnes, R. H. and Silvertsen, I. 1942. The Influence of Caloric Restriction Upon the Incidence of Spontaneous Mammary Carcinoma in Mice. Surgery. 1942; 11:48-55.

208. p. 123. Maugh, Thomas H. 1982. Cancer is not Inevitable. Science. 1982; 217:36-37.

209. p. 124. Dan, B., 1984. JAMA. 1984; 252:4.

210. p. 125. Sun, Marjorie, 1984. Biotechnology's Regulatory Tangle. Science. 1984; 225:697-698.

211. p. 126. Reif, Arnold E. 1975. Immunity and Cancer in Man: An Introduction. Immunology Series. Vol. III. Mallory Institute. Boston, Massachusetts. Publ. Marcel Deker, Inc. NY.

212. p. 126. Jausset, M. A. 1926. Diagnostic Value of Skin Reactions to Tuberculin in Adults. Accidental Surgery Bulletin. Mem. Soc. Hospital. Paris. 1926; 50:834-837.

213. p. 127. Bodey, Gerald P., Lerner, Martin A., Schemptf, Stephen. 1983. Gram Negative Infections. The Cancer Patient. Schering Co. Teaching Monograph. NY. 1983.

214. p. 128. Lewis, M. G., Hartman, D., and Jerry, L. M. 1976. Antibodies and Anti-Antibodies in Human Malignancy: An Expression of Deranged Immune Regulation. Annals NYAS. 1976; 276:316-327.

215. p. 130. Svet-Moldavsky, George J., Zinzar, Svetlana N., and Karmanova Natalia V. 1976. Inhibition of Tumor and Fetal Tissue Growth in Newborn Recipients. 1976. Annals. NYAS. 1976; 276:328-342.

216. p. 131. Davies, A. 1922. Lancet. 1922; 2:1009-1012.

217. p. 131. Ogra, P. L. 1969. The Secretory Immunologic System. Editors; D. H. Dayton, P. A. Small, R. M. Chanock, H. E. Kaufman, T. B. Tomasi. Nat. Inst. Child Health, Bethesda, Maryland. 1969. p. 259-279.

218. p. 131. Heremans, J. F., and Bazin H. 1971. antibodies Induced by Local Antigenic Stimulation of Mucosal Surfaces. Annals NYAS. 1971; 190:268-275.

219. p. 131, 132. Bellanti, Joseph, A. 1978. Immunology II Saunders Co. p. 399.

Chapter VII

220. p. 133. Cancer Basics. National Foundation for Cancer Research. 1984; 7 No. 1:1-2.

221. p. 133. Sypnosis of Activities. National Foundation for Cancer Research (NFCR). 1983. p.1 7315 Wisconsin Ave. Suite 332 Bethesda, Maryland 20814.

222. p. 134. Menneken, Hans L., MD, Unpublished Paper. St. Petersburg, FL 33707. (813) 345-4780.

223. p. 136. Brinkman, R., and Lamberts, H. B. 1958. Ozone as a Possible Radiomimetic Gas. Nature. 1958; 181:1202-1202.

224. p. 136. Teake, J. J., Badenburg, B., and Hoffman, W. 1973 Experimental Animal Studies on the Effect of Ozone on the Growth of Tumors and the Effect of Irradiation. 1973. Strahlentherapie. 1973; 145(2):155-160.

225. p. 136. Cotruvo, J. J., Simon, V. F. and Spanggord, R. J. 1977. Investigation of Mutagenic Effect of Products of Ozonations in Water. Annals. NYAS. 1977; 298:124-140.

226. p. 137. Rilling, S. 1983. The Possibilities of Medical Ozone Application in the Light of the Historical Developments of Ozone Therapy. Ozone News. Nachrichten Noveautes. 1983; 2:27-34.

227. p. 139. Sweet, Frederick, Ming-shian Koo, Song-Chiau D. Lee, Hagar, Will L., and Sweet, Nileen E. 1980. Ozone Selectively Inhibits Growth of Human Cancer Cells. Science. 1980; 209:931-933.

228. p. 146. Rokitansky, Otto. 1983. Clinical Study and Biochemistry of Ozone Therapy in Peripheral Arterial Circulatory Disorders. Paper presented in Washington DC at the Sixth Ozone World Congress of the International Ozone Association.

229. p. 1-7. Arnan, Migdalia. Effect of Ozone/Oxygen G Mixture Directly Injected Into the Mammary caecinoma of Female C3H/HEJ Mice. Paper was presented in Wash. DC. At the Sixth Ozone World Congress of the International Ozone association. This paper was published in 1985 in the Journal of Holistic Medicine. Vol. 7. NO. 1. Spring/Summer, 1985.

230. p. 149. Kervan, Louis C. 1872. Biological Transmutations. English Version. Michael Abehsera. Swan House Publishing Co. PO 170 Brooklyn, NY 11223. 1972. p. 49, 86, 115.

231. p. 150, 151. Szent-Gyorgi, Albert. 1984. Cancer Metabolism and Ascorbic Acid. Paper presented on September 17-18, 1984, in Washington DC at the International Symposium on Cancer Research.

---

232. p. 150. Becker, Robert O., and Marino, Andrew A. 1982. Electromagnetism of Life. State University of New York Press. Albany, NY. 1982. p. 21, 40, 41.

233. p. 151. March G., and Beams, H. W. 1952. Electrical Control of Morphogenesis in Regenerating Dugesia Tigrinum. J. Cell Comp. Physiol. 1952; 39:191.

234. p. 151. Humphrey and Seal, E. H. 1959. Biophysical Approach Toward Tumor Regression in Mice. Science. 1959; 130:388.

235. p. 153. Simone, Charles B. 1983. Cancer and Nutrition. McGraw-Hill Book Co. 1983.

Chapter VIII

236. p. 154 Eugene, H. and Schaeffer, Riley. Chemistry. 1973. Publ. Harper and Row. p. 237.

237. p. 156. Lehninger, Albert L. Second Edition. 1975. Worth Publishers Inc. 1975. p. 582-3.

238. p. 157. Watson, James D. 1976. Molecular Biology of the Gene. Third Edition. Publ. W. A. Benjamin, Inc. 1976. p. 582-3.

239. p. 157, 158. Bellanti, Joseph A. 1978. Immunology II. W. B. Saunders Company. 1978. p. 116-7.

240. p. 159. Kochwa, S., Terry, W. D., Capra, J. D., and Yang, N. L. 1971. Immunoglobulin E: Physicochemical Studies of the IgE Molecule, Annals NYAS. 1971; 190:49-70. p. 56.

241. p. 160. Davis, Bernard, and Dulbecco, Renato. 1970. Microbiology. Harper and Row. NY. Comparison of Chains of Immunoglobulins. p.432.

242. p. 160. Van Loghen, Erna. 1971. Formal Genetics of the Immunoglobulin System. Annals. NYAS. 1971; 190:136-149. p. 136.

243. p. 161.Sela, Michael. 1971. Effect of Antigenic structure on Antibody Biosynthesis. Annals NYAS. 1971; 190:181-202. p. 136.

244. p. 161. Edelman, Gerald M. 1959. Dissociation of Y-Globulins. 1959; 81:3155.

245. p. 161. Edelman, Gerald M. 1971. Antibody Structure and Molecular Immunology. Annals. NYAS. 1971; 190:5-25.

246. p. 161-164, 167. Burnet. Immunology Monograph. Scientific American. p. 27, 53, 54, 55, 76.

247. p. 169. Simpson, Robert W. 1976. Report to the Consumer. June, 1976. No. 127.

248. p. 170. Honorot, Ida, and McBean, E. 1977. Vaccination the Silent Killer. 1977. Honor Publications. PO Box 5449 Sherman Oaks, California 91403.

249. p. 171. Salk, Jonas, and Salk, Darrell. 1977. Science. March 4, 1977.

250. p. 171. Winter, Ruth. Cancer Causing Agents. A Preventive Guide. 1979. Crown Publ. Inc. NY.

251. p. 171. Sun, Marjorie. Compensation for Victims of Vaccines. 1981. Science. 1981; 211:906-908.

252. p. 172. Kurstak, R., and Kurstak, C. 1977. Comparative Diagnosis of Viral Disease. Vol. I. 1977. Academic Press, Inc.

253. p. 173. Family Practice Newa. December 1-14, 1984. p. 22.

254. p. 173. Trollforos. Acta Paediatr. Scan. 1984; 73:417-25.

255. p. 173. Sehon, A. H. 1982. Immunological Tolerance of the Self and Non-Self. Annals NYAS.1982; 392:55-70.

256. p. 173. Warren, Leonard, and Cossu, Giulio. 1982. The Bound Carbohydrates of the Glycoproteins in Normal and Pathological States. Annals NYAS. Endothelium. 1982; 401:86.

257. p. 173. Megaw and Johnson. 1979. Glycoproteins Synthesized by Cultures Cells; Effect of Serum Concentrations and Buffers on Sugar Content. Proc. Soc. Exp. Biol. Med. 1979; 161:60-65.

258. p. 174. Traskalova-Hogenova, H., Sterzl, J., et al. 1983. The Development of Immunological Capacity Under Germfree and Conventional Conditions. The Excretory Immune System. Annals. NYAS. 1983; 409:580-592.

259. p. 174. Leffler, H., Lomberg, H., Botschlich, E., Jodal, U., Korhonen, K., Samuelsson, B. E., Schoolnik, G., and Svanborg, Eden C. 1982. Chemical and Clinical Studies on the Interaction of E. coli With Host Glycolipids Receptors in Urinary Tract Infection. Scan. J. Dis. Suppl. 1982; 833:26-32.

Chapter IX

260. p. 176. Notkins and Koprowoski. 1973. How the Immune Response to a Virus Can Cause Disease. Scientific American. Immunology Monograph. January 1973.

261. p. 176. Rowe, Wallace P. 1950. Virus Effect on Coriomeningitis. Scientific American Monograph in Immunology.

262. p. 180. Stern, Richard. 1984. Managing Pain and Presenting Symptom. October 1984.

263. p. 181, 182. Kurstack R., and Kurstack, C. 1977. Comparative Diagnosis of Viral Disease. Vol. I. 1977. Academic Press Inc.

264. p. 182. Greaces, F. M., Rickson, A. B. 1975. Clin. Immunopathol. 1975; 3:514-524.

265. p. 182. Reedman, B. M., and Klein, G. 1973. Int. J. Cancer. 1973; 11:499-520.

266. p. 183. Kurstak, R., and Kurtak, C. Comparative Diagnosis of Viral Diseases. Vol. II. 1977. p. 115.

267. p. 183. Temin, H. M., and Mitzutani, S. 1970. Nature. 1970; 226:1121-1123.

268. p. 183. Baltimore, D. 1970. Nature. 1970; 226:1209-1211.

269. p. 185. Marx, Jean L. 1982. Cancer Cell Genes Linked to Viral Oncogenes. Science. 1982; 216:724.

270. p. 185. Huebner, R. J., and Tadaro, G. J. 1969. Proc. Natl. Acad. Sci. USA. 1969; 64:1087-1094.

271. p. 186. Yasushi Ono, et al. 1974. Monograph on Cancer Immunology #16. University of Tokyo Press. p. 37.

272. p. 186. Orita, K., et al. 1974. Monograph Cancer Research #16. University of Tokyo Press. p. 37.

273. p. 186. Kikuchi, K., et al. 1974. Tumor-Specific Cell-Mediated Immune Reactions. Cancer Immunology Monograph #16. University. of Tokyo Press. Japan. 1974. p. 109.

274. p. 187. Lewis et al. 1976. Antibodies and Anti-Antibodies in Human Malignancy: An Expression of Deranged Immune Regulation. Annals NYAS. 1976; 276:316-327.

275. p. 189. Jerne. Ciba Symposium. 1972

Chapter 10.

276. Dr. Hyman, M. and Liponis, M. "Ultra-Prevention" . Book. 2005

277. Dr. Hyman, M. "Ultrametabolism". Book. 2008

278. Kaufmann, Doug A. "The Fungus Link". Books. 2000-2008

279. Dr. Braverman, Eric R. "Younger You (Thinner) You Diet". Book 2009

280. Dr. Leaf, Caroline. "The Gift in You". Book. 2009

281. The Silva Life System. Meditation. The Silva Method.

282. Dr. Leaf. Caroline. "Who Switched Off my Brain?". Book. 1982

283. Hemmes, Hilde. "The Traditional Uses of Herbs." Book. 1999

CPSIA information can be obtained
at www.ICGtesting.com
Printed in the USA
BVHW030708160721
611876BV00014B/40/J